FIBROM NUT

MW01289261

A SAFE AND EFFECTIVE FUNCTIONAL MEDICINE STRATEGY

DR. ALEX VASQUEZ

- Doctor of Osteopathic Medicine, graduate of University of North Texas Health Science Center, Texas College of Osteopathic Medicine (2010)
- Doctor of Naturopathic Medicine, graduate of Bastyr University (1999)
- Doctor of Chiropractic, graduate of Western States Chiropractic College (1996)
- Director of the Medical Board of Advisors (2011-present), Researcher and Lecturer (2004-2010), Biotics Research Corporation in Rosenberg, Texas
- Adjunct Faculty (2004-2005, 2010-present) and Forum Consultant (2003-2007), The Institute for Functional Medicine in Gig Harbor, Washington
- Program Director for Master of Science in Nutrition and Functional Medicine, University of Western States in Portland, Oregon
- Former Adjunct Professor of Orthopedics (2000) and Rheumatology (2001), Bastyr University in Kenmore, Washington
- Private practice in Seattle, Washington (2000-2001), Houston, Texas (2001-2006), Portland, Oregon (2011-present)
- Author of approximately 100 articles and letters published in *Annals of Pharmacotherapy, The Lancet, Nutritional Perspectives, BMJ—British Medical Journal, Journal of Manipulative and Physiological Therapeutics, JAMA—Journal of the American Medical Association, The Original Internist, Integrative Medicine, Holistic Primary Care, Nutritional Wellness, Dynamic Chiropractic, Alternative Therapies in Health and Medicine, JAOA—Journal of the American Osteopathic Association, Evidence-based Complementary and Alternative Medicine, Journal of Clinical Endocrinology and Metabolism*, and *Arthritis & Rheumatism*: Official Journal of the American College of Rheumatology

OPTIMALHEALTHRESEARCH.COM

Vasquez A. <u>Fibromyalgia in a Nutshell: A Safe and Effective Functional Medicine Strategy</u>. Portland, Oregon; Integrative and Biological Medicine Research and Consulting, LLC.

The intended audiences for this book are health science students and doctorate-level clinicians. This book has been written with every intention to make it as accurate as possible, and each section has undergone peer-review by an interdisciplinary group of clinicians. In view of the possibility of human error and as well as ongoing discoveries in the biomedical sciences, neither the author nor any party associated in any way with this text warrants that this text is perfect, accurate, or complete in every way, and we disclaim responsibility for harm or loss associated with the application of the material herein. Information and treatments applicable to a specific *condition* may not be appropriate for or applicable to a specific *patient*; this is especially true for patients with multiple comorbidities and those taking pharmaceutical medications with multiple adverse effects and drug/nutrient/herb interactions. Given that this book is available on an open market, lay persons who read this material should discuss the information with a licensed healthcare provider before implementing any treatments and interventions described herein.

See website for updated information: www.OptimalHealthResearch.com

Dedications: I dedicate this book to the following people in appreciation for their works, their direct and indirect support of this work, and for their contributions to the advancement of true healthcare.

- **To the students and practitioners of chiropractic and naturopathic medicine**, those who continue to learn so that they can provide the best possible care to their patients.
- **To the researchers** whose works are cited in this text.
- **To Drs Alan Gaby, Jeffrey Bland, Ronald LeFebvre, Robert Richard, and Gilbert Manso,** my most memorable and influential professors and mentors.
- **To Dr Bruce Ames**[1] **and the late Dr Roger Williams**[2], for helping us to view our individuality as biochemically unique.
- **To Dr Chester Wilk**[3,4] **and important others** for documenting and resisting the organized oppression of natural, non-pharmaceutical, non-surgical healthcare.[5,6,7]
- **To Jorge Strunz and Ardeshir Farah,** for artistic inspiration

Acknowledgments for Peer and Editorial Review: Acknowledgement here does not imply that the reviewer fully agrees with or endorses the material in this text but rather that they were willing to review specific sections of the book for clinical applicability and clarity and to make suggestions to their own level of satisfaction. Credit for improvements and refinements to this text are due in part to these reviewers; responsibility for oversights remains that of the author.

- 2012 Edition of Fibromyalgia in a Nutshell: Lisa Scholl BA, Annette D'Armatta ND
- 2012 Edition of Migraine Headaches, Hypothyroidism, and Fibromyalgia: Holly Furlong DC
- 2011 Edition of *Integrative Chiropractic Management of High Blood Pressure and Chronic Hypertension*: Barry Morgan MD, Holly Furlong DC, Kris Young DC, Erika Mennerick DC, and Bill Beakey DOM
- 2011 Edition of *Integrative Medicine and Functional Medicine for Chronic Hypertension*: Erika Mennerick DC, Holly Furlong DC, JoAnn Fawcett DC, Ileana Bourland MSOM LAc, James Bogash DC, Bill Beakey
- 2010 Edition of *Chiropractic Management of Chronic Hypertension*: Joseph Paun MS DC, Joe Brimhall DC, David Candelario OMS4 (TCOM c/o 2010), James Bogash DC, Bill Beakey DOM, Robert Richard DO
- 2009 Edition of *Chiropractic and Naturopathic Mastery of Common Clinical Disorders*: Heather Kahn MD, Robert Richard DO, James Leiber DO, David Candelario (UNT-HSC TCOM DO4)
- 2007 Edition of *Integrative Orthopedics*: Barry Morgan MD, Dennis Harris DC, Richard Brown DC (DACBI candidate), Ron Mariotti ND, Patrick Makarewich MBA, Reena Singh (SCNM ND4), Zachary Watkins DC, Charles Novak MS DC, Marnie Loomis ND, James Bogash DC, Sara Croteau DC, Kris Young DC, Joshua Levitt ND, Jack Powell III MD, Chad Kessler MD, Amy Neuzil ND
- 2006 Edition of *Integrative Rheumatology*: Amy Neuzil ND, Cathryn Harbor MD, Julian Vickers DC, Tamara Sachs MD, Bob Sager BSc MD DABFM (Clinical Instructor in the Department of Family Medicine, University of Kansas), Ron Mariotti ND, Titus Chiu (DC4), Zachary Watkins (DC4), Gilbert Manso MD, Bruce Milliman ND, William Groskopp DC, Robert Silverman DC, Matthew Breske (DC4), Dean Neary ND, Thomas Walton DC, Fraser Smith ND, Ladd Carlston DC, David Jones MD, Joshua Levitt ND
- 2004 Edition of *Integrative Orthopedics*: Peter Knight ND, Kent Littleton ND MS, Barry Morgan MD, Ron Hobbs ND, Joshua Levitt ND, John Neustadt (Bastyr ND4), Allison Gandre BS (Bastyr ND4), Peter Kimble ND, Jack Powell III MD, Chad Kessler MD, Mike Gruber MD, Deirdre O'Neill ND, Mary Webb ND, Leslie Charles ND, Amy Neuzil ND

Fibromyalgia

Introduction:

Fibromyalgia—also referred to as fibromyalgia syndrome (FMS)—is a clinical entity that has remained enigmatic to the medical profession despite the consistent publication of research that delineates its cause and its effective treatments. This chapter summarizes clinical assessments, treatments, and essential background information that should provide empowering knowledge for clinicians and for the patients suffering with this condition.

<u>Topics</u>:

- Introduction and Overview
- Clinical Presentation
- Prevalence, symptoms, and clinical findings
- Pathophysiology
- Diagnosis
- Standard Medical Treatment for Fibromyalgia
- Functional Medicine Considerations, Assessments, and Interventions
- Conditions that Mimic or Contribute to Symptoms of Fibromyalgia
- Small intestine bacterial overgrowth (SIBO) as the ultimate cause of and most logical explanation for FM
- Therapeutic Interventions
- Conclusions and Clinical Approach

Fibromyalgia (FM)

Introduction

- **Overview**: Fibromyalgia (FM) is commonly described as an "idiopathic" (of unknown origin) syndrome principally characterized by widespread body pain and numerous myofascial tender points at specific locations. FM is most common in women 20-50 years of age, and the condition often presents with associated complaints of fatigue, headaches, subjective numbness, altered sleep patterns, and gastrointestinal disturbances. FM in children and adolescents presents similarly to FM in adults except for the comparatively higher prevalence of sleep disturbance and the finding of fewer tender points in children.[8] Until recently, fibromyalgia was considered a *diagnosis of exclusion* after infection, autoimmunity, or other primary causes of widespread pain were excluded by clinical and laboratory assessment. However, current criteria base the diagnosis on positive findings of chronic, widespread musculoskeletal pain in characteristic locations; these criteria will be described below. Fibromyalgia shares several clinical, demographic, and pathologic features with chronic fatigue syndrome (CFS) and irritable bowel syndrome (IBS); the reason for these overlaps is not generally understood by most clinicians and researchers but will be made plain in this writing.
- **The common medical view—scientifically inaccurate, financially leveraged**: The prevailing medical view, expressed by most medical doctors and the authors of widely cited articles, is that fibromyalgia is idiopathic—*of unknown origin*—with strong neuropsychogenic (*neuro*=nerves and brain, *psyche*=mind, *genic*=origin) influences (in other words, "It's all in your head.") and that, since the underlying causes of the condition have not been identified, the best therapeutic approach is symptom suppression via perpetual pharmacotherapy with adjunctive use of psychotherapy and limited exercise.[9,10,11] This prevailing medical view is unscientific (not based on science) and counterscientific (ignores and contradicts published and validated research), unethical (fails to provide effective treatment when such treatment is available; condemns patients to medicalization and suffering), and commercially leveraged (diagnostic criteria revision and many review articles discussing treatment are sponsored by drug companies; medical profession benefits financially by having many long-term drug-dependent patients).
- **Fibromyalgia is a disease, not a syndrome**: The term *syndrome* connotes that a cluster of symptoms is of a nonorganic, psychogenic, or idiopathic nature, whereas *disease* validates the organic and pathophysiological nature of an illness. This author advocates the use of *disease* rather than *syndrome*

when describing fibromyalgia in appreciation of the real, organic, biochemical, and histopathological (*histo*=cells and tissues, *pathological*=disease) findings which clearly indicate that fibromyalgia is a specific disease entity and not simply a psychogenic or enigmatic cluster of symptoms. If fibromyalgia is a real, organic clinical entity (as will be documented here), then the appropriate designation is *fibromyalgia disease* (FMD) rather than *fibromyalgia syndrome* (FMS). For consistency and clarity within this section, the general term "fibromyalgia" will be used. Relatedly, the term "irritable bowel syndrome" (IBS) is also a misnomer that confuses professionals as well as the general public into thinking that the condition does not have identified causes and (nonpharmaceutical) treatments; despite promulgations to the contrary, the cause of IBS is well-known[12], and effective treatment is readily available.

Clinical Presentation

- **Prevalence, symptoms, and clinical findings**: Fibromyalgia is one of the most common chronic pain conditions, affecting an estimated 10 million people in the U.S. and an estimated 3-6% of people world-wide.[13] Approximately 10% of affected patients have severe symptoms resulting in partial or total disability. Affected patients report chronic aches, pains, and stiffness with a proclivity for localization near the neck, shoulders, low back, and hips. Pain and fatigue are typically exacerbated following physical exertion or psychological stress. Associated manifestations include fatigue, sleep disorders (including insomnia, unrefreshing sleep, and objective abnormalities such as an increase in stage 1 sleep, a reduction in delta sleep, and alpha-delta sleep anomaly), subjective numbness, headaches, and gastrointestinal disturbances consistent with a clinical diagnosis of irritable bowel syndrome (IBS). Clinical findings shared between FM and IBS include abdominal pain and discomfort, changed frequency of stool, diarrhea and/or constipation, abdominal bloating/distention/gas and flatulence, dyspepsia/heartburn, headaches especially migraine-type headaches), fatigue, myalgias, restless leg syndrome, anxiety, and depression. The **high prevalence (>50%) of migraine-type headaches in FM patients** suggests an underlying pathogenesis shared between cephalgia (*ceph*=head, *algia*=pain) and widespread myalgia (*myo*=muscle, *algia*=pain); one of the established and most likely causative abnormalities shared between migraine and FM is impaired mitochondrial function, which will be explained in greater detail later in this publication. Cognitive symptoms such as "brain fog" ("fibro-fog") and difficulty with memory and word retrieval, as well as **environmental intolerance (EI) and multiple chemical sensitivity (MCS),** are seen in both FM and CFS[14]; again, this overlap of shared symptoms suggests a common etiopathogenesis (*etio*=cause, *patho*=disease, *genesis*=initiation). Routine physical examination and laboratory findings are generally normal, with the exception the physical examination finding of fibromyalgia tender points (described and diagrammed below in the section on Diagnosis per the 1990 diagnostic criteria).

Pathophysiology

- **Abnormalities noted in muscle tissue of patients with FM**: Muscle biopsies from patients with fibromyalgia show numerous histological, ultrastructural, and biochemical abnormalities, including defects in mitochondrial structure and function, reduced numbers of capillaries in skeletal muscle (leading to reduced blood supply to muscles), thickened capillary endothelium (thicker vessel walls), and ragged red fibers consistent with the development of **mitochondrial myopathy** (*myo*=muscle, *pathos*=disease). The histological finding of "rubber-band morphology" with reticular threads connecting neighboring cells in muscle biopsies of FM patients is associated with prolonged contractions in adjacent/neighboring muscle fibers; these abnormalities result in and perpetuate a low-energy state within myocytes (*myo*=muscle, *cytes*=cells).[15] Other studies have shown disorganization of actin filaments, accumulation of lipofuscin (cellular debris) consistent with premature muscle aging, accumulation of glycogen and lipid accumulation consistent with **mitochondrial impairment**, increased DNA fragmentation, **significant reductions in the number of mitochondria**, and focal areas of chronic muscle contraction.[16] These histological abnormalities are important and establish the fact that **fibromyalgia is a *disease of metabolic dysfunction*** rather than an *emotional disorder of psychogenic origin*; therefore, attributing the pain and fatigue of fibromyalgia to a mental-psychological cause or a central nervous system disorder such as central sensitization is unscientific and illogical.

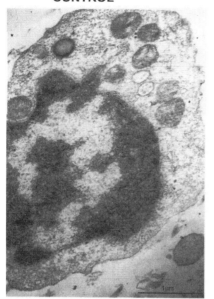
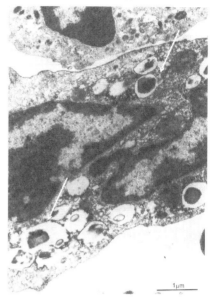

Blood cells in FM patients show mitochondrial destruction (mitophagy), as well as smaller size and lower number of mitochondria, indicating impaired mitochondrial function and reduced energy production: Structure of blood mononuclear cells (BMCs, cells of the immune system) from FM patients. The healthy/control BMCs show mitochondria with a normal structure. Autophagosomes (indicated by arrows), where mitochondria are destroyed (the process of mitophagy [*mito*=mitochondria, *phagy*=consumption], are noted in the BMCs of patients with FM. [Bar = 1 micrometer]. This open-access image is respectfully attributed to the brilliant research published by these researchers Cordero MD, De Miguel M, Moreno Fernández AM, Carmona López IM, Garrido Maraver J, Cotán D, Gómez Izquierdo L, Bonal P, Campa F, Bullon P, Navas P, Sánchez Alcázar JA. Mitochondrial dysfunction and mitophagy activation in blood mononuclear cells of fibromyalgia patients: implications in the pathogenesis of the disease. *Arthritis Res Ther.* 2010;12(1):R17 http://arthritis-research.com/content/12/1/R17

- **Biochemical abnormalities noted in patients with FM**: Ultrastructural and biochemical abnormalities appear to be more pathologically significant and clinically relevant than the noted histological changes in skeletal muscle biopsy samples. Importantly, **the biochemical abnormalities *are the cause* of the histologic/tissue abnormalities**. Numerous **mitochondrial enzyme defects are seen**, including reduced activity of 3-hydroxy-CoA dehydrogenase, citrate synthase, and cytochrome oxidase. Levels of free magnesium are reduced by 31%, and levels of complexed ATP-magnesium are reduced by 12% in muscle from FM patients compared with levels seen in healthy controls; these biochemical and bioenergetic defects contribute to rapid-onset fatigue and muscle pain. From a neurophysiological perspective, magnesium can promote hypersensitivity to pain due to a reduction in the partial blockade of N-methyl-D-aspartate (NMDA) neurotransmitter receptor sites.[17] Reduced perfusion of muscle tissue during exercise results in relative tissue hypoxia, reduced muscle healing after the microtrauma of exercise, and promotion of muscle soreness due to accumulation of L-lactate (lactic acid).[18] **Increased oxidative stress** is also seen in FM patients,[19] providing additional objective evidence of the systemic, organic, and non-psychogenic nature of the illness. Evidence of hypothalamic-pituitary-adrenal disturbance and **increased cytokine production (particularly interleukin-8, which promotes sympathetic pain, and interleukin-6, which induces hyperalgesia [increased perception of pain], fatigue, and depression**[20]) further characterize the systemic and organic nature of this condition and are well documented in the research literature. **The majority of fibromyalgia patients demonstrate laboratory evidence of bacterial overgrowth in the small bowel**[21], and the details and important implications of this will be discussed below. **Vitamin D deficiency**—a recognized cause of chronic widespread pain as well as depression, muscle fatigue, and chronic low-grade inflammation—is also common in fibromyalgia patients.[22,23] FM patients have **significantly elevated blood levels of pentosidine**, which is an advanced glycation end-product (AGE) which is a marker of oxidative stress and glycosylation (sugar-protein binding); AGEs promote chronic inflammation and sensitization leading to chronic pain.[24] Another AGE very similar to pentosidine, **carboxy-methyl-lysine (CML) is found in higher levels in the blood and muscle of FM patients**[25]; both pentosidine and CML cause expedited "muscle aging" and promote chronic pain and inflammation. These objective abnormalities of biochemical, histological, nutritional, and microbiological/gastrointestinal status force clinicians to appreciate the valid and organic nature of fibromyalgia. As previously stated, this evidence refutes promulgations espoused within standard allopathic/pharmaceutical medicine that fibromyalgia is an idiopathic condition warranting lifelong medicalization with expensive and potentially hazardous analgesic and antidepressant drugs; the focus on drug treatment to mask/suppress the pain of fibromyalgia detours doctors and patients away from focusing on the treatable causes of fibromyalgia pain.

Objective "organic" abnormalities noted in patients with fibromyalgia
1. Histologic and functional abnormalities in muscle tissue: Disorganization of actin filaments, accumulation of lipofuscin bodies consistent with premature muscle aging, increased DNA fragmentation, and focal areas of chronic muscle contraction, reduced perfusion of muscle tissue during exercise (i.e., reduced blood flow to muscles).
2. Mitochondrial defects: Accumulation of glycogen (muscle sugar) and lipid (fat) indicate that intracellular energy production is impaired and that the cells are unable to efficiently convert fuel sources into energy in the form of ATP, adenosine triphosphate, which is the basic fuel source for cellular metabolism. Also noted are significant reductions in the number of mitochondria, reduced activity of important enzymes such as 3-hydroxy-CoA dehydrogenase, citrate synthase, and cytochrome oxidase. Nutritional deficiencies, such as CoQ-10 deficiency, promote mitochondrial dysfunction, thus leading to mitochondrial destruction (mitophagy) which ultimately results in reduced numbers of mitochondria and perpetuates and aggravates muscle fatigue, pain, and neurocognitive dysfunction (i.e., brain fog, difficulty thinking, depression).
3. Oxidative stress: Increased oxidative stress results from mitochondrial dysfunction and nutrient depletion.
4. Neuroendocrine abnormalities: Hypothalamic-pituitary-adrenal (HPA) disturbance indicates impaired function of the brain and endocrine system.
5. Low-grade immune activation: Increased cytokine production indicates a pro-inflammatory state.
6. Bacterial overgrowth in the intestines: FM patients nearly always have excess/overgrowth of bacteria in their intestines, referred to as SIBO—small intestine bacterial overgrowth.
7. High prevalence of vitamin D deficiency: Common in the general population but more common in patients with chronic pain; vitamin D deficiency causes chronic pain, depression/anxiety, and low-grade inflammation—all of these problems are seen in patients with fibromyalgia.
8. Low blood levels of L-tryptophan: FM patients have low levels of the amino acid tryptophan in their blood, despite adequate dietary intake. The most likely explanation for the deficiency of tryptophan is destruction of tryptophan by bacterial enzyme action. Several intestinal bacteria produce the enzyme tryptophanase, which destroys the amino acid tryptophan. Bacterial overgrowth results in more tryptophanase, resulting in tryptophan deficiency. Deficiency of tryptophan results in deficiencies of the hormones serotonin and melatonin, which result in anxiety, depression, food/sugar cravings, unrestful sleep, and mitochondrial dysfunction, since deficiency of melatonin causes reduced mitochondrial energy-production efficiency.

Diagnosis

- **Clinical criteria—description and contrast of the 1990 criteria and the 2010 criteria**: Per guidelines published in 1990 by the American College of Rheumatology (ACR), a diagnosis of fibromyalgia can be made in a patient with inexplicable, widespread myofascial pain of at least 3 months' duration; *inexplicable* denotes normalcy of routine laboratory and physical examination findings and failure to find an alternate explanation or diagnosis, while *widespread* denotes bilateral pain above and below the waist not attributable to trauma or rheumatic disease and with pain at 11 of

18 classic tender point locations (see illustration below). FM tender points are assessed bilaterally at 9 paired sites: (sub)occiput (below the head at the neckline), low cervical spine (lower neck), trapezius and supraspinatus (two of the shoulder muscles), second rib (anterior, near costosternal [rib-breastbone] junction), lateral epicondyle, gluteal region, greater trochanter, and medial fat pad of the knees. Tender points are provoked by the clinician's application of approximately 9 pounds of fingertip pressure, which is sufficient to cause blanching of the clinician's nail bed. The tender points of fibromyalgia are distinguished from myofascial trigger points (MFTP, described by Travell[26]) and strain-counterstrain tender points (described in the osteopathic literature by Jones[27]). In contrast to MFTP, which are located toward the center of the muscle fiber and which refer pain and show spontaneous electrocontractile activity[28], tender points of fibromyalgia are located near the tendinous insertions of muscle to bone and cause local pain only, without pain referral or contractile activity.

Illustration showing the 9 paired locations of fibromyalgia tender points:
Per the 1990 ACR guidelines, the diagnosis of fibromyalgia is supported when at least 11 out of 18 of these locations are painful.

Clinical findings: Pain, on digital palpation, must be present in at least 11 of the following 18 tender point sites:

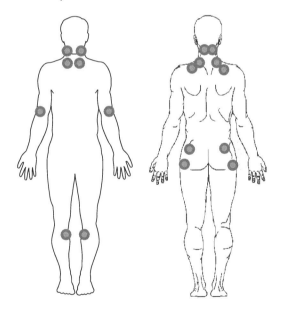

1. Occiput: at the suboccipital muscle insertions.
2. Low cervical: at the anterior aspects of the intertransverse spaces at C5-C7.
3. Trapezius: at the midpoint of the upper border.
4. Supraspinatus: at origins, above the scapula spine near the medial border.
5. Second rib: upper lateral to the second costochondral junction.
6. Lateral epicondyle: 2 cm distal to the epicondyles.
7. Gluteal: in upper outer quadrants of buttocks in anterior fold of muscle.
8. Greater trochanter: posterior to the trochanteric prominence.
9. Knee: at the medial fat pad proximal to the joint line.

Digital palpation should be performed with an approximate force of 4 kg (9 lbs). A tender point has to be painful at palpation, not just "tender."[29]

In 2010, new ACR guidelines for the diagnosis and assessment of FM[30] were significantly changed from the 1990 guidelines. Very curiously, the authors state that one of their objectives was to create criteria that "do not require a tender point examination"; at first, this seems odd and clinically inconsistent considering that the tender point examination ❶ takes only about 60 seconds to perform, ❷ is noninvasive, ❸ was previously the standard by which the diagnosis was made, and ❹ is reasonable and responsible—physical examination of patients with pain is a reasonable standard of care. Oddly, the authors of the new guidelines note several "important problems" with the 1990 ACR criteria, such as "Patients who improved or whose symptoms and tender points decreased could fail to satisfy the ACR 1990 classification definition" and "there was little variation in symptoms among fibromyalgia patients." Clinicians should note that these so-called "problems" *are not problems at all* because patients who improve and thus no longer meet diagnostic criteria should not be considered to have an active disease/diagnosis, and that high-quality clinical criteria should indeed result in the specific definition of clinical disorder and thus in a well-defined cohort of patients; correcting these "problems" results in patients being diagnosed for longer periods of time (more *long-term* patients) and also results in more patients being diagnosed with fibromyalgia (more *total* patients). Perhaps even more curious is the fact that development of these new guidelines was sponsored by Lilly Research Laboratories, which is the "research" section of Eli Lilly and Company, one of the world's largest drug companies and the manufacturer of duloxetine/Cymbalta® which is one of the only drugs approved by the US Food and Drug Administration (FDA) for the treatment of fibromyalgia.[31] Among patients labeled with fibromyalgia, the new criteria increase the percentage of patients diagnosable by criteria from 75% to 88%; whether the motivation to expand the patient population diagnosed with fibromyalgia is altruistic or financially motivated is subject to debate.

The new criteria rely on a summation of two tallies—"widespread pain index" (WPI) and "symptom severity" (SS, parts 1 and 2)—with the diagnosis being supported by either **"WPI >7 and SS >5"** or **"WPI 3–6 and SS >9"**. Pain must have been consistent for at least three months and must not be attributable to another (obvious) cause.

2010 Fibromyalgia diagnostic criteria—summary and chart for clinical use

Widespread pain index (WPI): each positive location receives one point (max = 19)

1. Shoulder girdle, left	7. Hip (buttock/trochanter), left	13. Jaw, left
2. Shoulder girdle, right	8. Hip (buttock/trochanter), right	14. Jaw, right
3. Upper arm, left	9. Upper leg, left	15. Chest (sternum area)
4. Upper arm, right	10. Upper leg, right	16. Abdomen
5. Lower arm, left	11. Lower leg, left	17. Neck
6. Lower arm, right	12. Lower leg, right	18. Upper back
		19. Lower back

Symptom severity (SS)—part 1: Each of the following three problems is quantified with the following scale (total max = 9):

    0 none: no problem
    1 mild: intermittent or mild problems
    2 moderate: often present, considerable problems
    3 severe: pervasive, continuous, life-disturbing problems

0 1 2 3　Fatigue	0 1 2 3　Waking unrefreshed	0 1 2 3　Cognitive symptoms

Symptom severity (SS)—part 2: The clinician considers the patient's "somatic symptoms in general" (listed below) and applies the following scale (max = 3):

    0 no symptoms
    1 few symptoms
    2 a moderate number of symptoms
    3 a great deal of symptoms

0 1 2 3　muscle pain	0 1 2 3　itching	
0 1 2 3　irritable bowel syndrome	0 1 2 3　wheezing	
0 1 2 3　fatigue/tiredness	0 1 2 3　Raynaud's phenomenon	
0 1 2 3　thinking or remembering problems	0 1 2 3　hives/welts	
0 1 2 3　muscle weakness	0 1 2 3　ringing in ears	
0 1 2 3　headache	0 1 2 3　vomiting	
0 1 2 3　pain/cramps in the abdomen	0 1 2 3　heartburn	
0 1 2 3　numbness/tingling	0 1 2 3　oral ulcers	
0 1 2 3　dizziness	0 1 2 3　loss of/change in taste	
0 1 2 3　insomnia	0 1 2 3　seizures	
0 1 2 3　depression	0 1 2 3　dry eyes	
0 1 2 3　constipation	0 1 2 3　shortness of breath	
0 1 2 3　pain in the upper abdomen	0 1 2 3　loss of appetite	
0 1 2 3　nausea	0 1 2 3　skin rash	
0 1 2 3　nervousness	0 1 2 3　sun sensitivity	
0 1 2 3　chest pain	0 1 2 3　hearing difficulties	
0 1 2 3　blurred vision	0 1 2 3　easy bruising	
0 1 2 3　fever	0 1 2 3　hair loss	
0 1 2 3　diarrhea	0 1 2 3　frequent urination	
0 1 2 3　dry mouth	0 1 2 3　painful urination	
	0 1 2 3　bladder spasms	

Patients may be diagnosed with fibromyalgia if "WPI >7 and SS >5" or "WPI 3–6 and SS >9".

Tally from above:　WPI = _____
                        SS1 = _____
                        SS2 = _____
                    Total = _____

- **Clinical profile and findings on common laboratory tests**: New-onset fibromyalgia is unlikely over age 50, and the condition never causes fever, significant weight loss, or other objective signs of acute or subacute illness. Hypothyroidism is common and can produce widespread myofascial pain along with depression and other complaints, resulting in a clinical picture that closely resembles FM; thus, a complete thyroid evaluation (detailed later) is essential during the initial evaluation of any fibromyalgia-like condition. Common rheumatic conditions such as rheumatoid arthritis (RA) and systemic lupus erythematosus (SLE) are excluded by the lack of other clinical manifestations (e.g., joint pain and swelling) and the lack of positive laboratory findings such as anti-cyclic citrullinated protein (CCP) antibodies and antinuclear antibodies (ANA), respectively. C-reactive protein (CRP) and erythrocyte sedimentation rate (ESR) are normal in FM patients; abnormalities with these or other common laboratory assessments suggest inflammatory disease, infection, or other concomitant illness. Hypophosphatemia (a low level of the electrolyte phosphate in the blood) can cause bone pain and muscle weakness; this condition is easily excluded by demonstration of normal serum phosphate level.

Standard Medical Treatment for Fibromyalgia
- **Overview**: Mild exercise, "patient education", and the use of pain-relieving drugs are mainstays of standard medical treatment delivered by most allopathic medical doctors (MDs), and osteopathic medical doctors (DOs) may add manual musculoskeletal treatments to enhance the benefits of drugs.[32] These interventions are only partially effective and offer no hope of actually curing the disease; thus, medical treatment relegates patients to a future of drug dependency, potential adverse effects (some of which can be fatal), and therapeutic inefficacy insofar as none of these treatments addresses the underlying cause of the disorder.
  - **Amitriptyline**: For many years, the most widely used drug for symptomatic treatment of fibromyalgia was amitriptyline (a tricyclic antidepressant), which has been used "off label"—without approval from the FDA—for this application. In the treatment of FM, the drug has low efficacy and high potential for adverse effects; up to 20% of patients suffer from weight gain, constipation, orthostatic hypotension, and/or agitation as a side-effect of the drug. Only 25% to 30% of fibromyalgia patients experience clinically significant improvement with amitriptyline.[33] According to recent research in rats, administration of amitriptyline causes deficiency of CoQ-10, impaired mitochondrial function, reduced ATP/energy production, and increased oxidative stress and free radical damage[34]; all of these drug-

induced problems (discussed in detail later in this paper) are expected to worsen the pain and suffering experienced by FM patients. Thus, the use of amitriptyline cannot be considered to be consistent with the practice of good medicine due to its low efficacy and unacceptable risks for adverse effects.

o **Pregabalin**: In 2007, the United States Food and Drug Administration (US FDA) approved pregabalin (Lyrica® sold/marketed by Pfizer) for symptomatic treatment of fibromyalgia[35]; however, because the drug does not address the primary cause(s) of the disease, patients must continue treatment indefinitely. Adverse effects of pregabalin include dizziness, sleepiness, blurred vision, **weight gain**, dry mouth, swelling of hands and feet, impairment of motor function, and problems with concentration and attention. Pregabalin when given at the recommended dose of 150-225 mg twice per day for fibromyalgia costs $94-190 per month (pricing in 2012).

Suicide and depression risk warning for pregabalin/Lyrica from the US FDA
"Antiepileptics drugs (AEDs), including Lyrica, increase the risk of suicidal thoughts or behavior in patients taking these drugs for any indication. Patients treated with any AED for any indication should be monitored for the emergence or worsening of depression, suicidal thoughts or behavior, and/or any unusual changes in mood or behavior."
http://www.fda.gov/Safety/MedWatch/SafetyInformation /Safety-RelatedDrugLabelingChanges/ucm154524.htm Accessed September 2012

o **Duloxetine**: In 2008, the FDA announced duloxetine (Cymbalta® sold/marketed by Lilly) as the second approved drug for the treatment of fibromyalgia. Ironically, many physicians consider any "approved" drug to have scientific substantiation; however, in the case of duloxetine (as well as pregabalin) the exact mechanism of action is unknown[36] although duloxetine appears to inhibit reuptake of norepinephrine and serotonin, thereby increasing the action of these neurotransmitters in the synaptic cleft. Adverse effects from duloxetine include nausea, dry mouth, sleepiness, constipation, decreased appetite, and increased sweating; **duloxetine can also increase the risk of suicidal thinking and behavior and for this reason the drug carries a black box warning on the container**. Duloxetine can cause serious and fatal adverse effects including the following: worsening depression and suicidality, serotonin syndrome, neuroleptic malignant syndrome, seizures, and Stevens-Johnson syndrome. Duloxetine given at the recommended dose of 60 mg per day for FM costs $170 per month (pricing in 2012).

Black box warning for duloxetine/Cymbalta

"WARNING: Suicidality and Antidepressant Drugs: Antidepressants increased the risk compared to placebo of suicidal thinking and behavior (suicidality) in children, adolescents, and young adults in short-term studies of major depressive disorder (MDD) and other psychiatric disorders. Anyone considering the use of Cymbalta or any other antidepressant in a child, adolescent, or young adult must balance this risk with the clinical need. Short-term studies did not show an increase in the risk of suicidality with antidepressants compared to placebo in adults beyond age 24; there was a reduction in risk with antidepressants compared to placebo in adults aged 65 and older. Depression and certain other psychiatric disorders are themselves associated with increases in the risk of suicide. Patients of all ages who are started on antidepressant therapy should be monitored appropriately and observed closely for clinical worsening, suicidality, or unusual changes in behavior. Families and caregivers should be advised of the need for close observation and communication with the prescriber. Cymbalta is not approved for use in pediatric patients."

http://pi.lilly.com/us/cymbalta-pi.pdf Accessed January 2012

- o **Milnacipran**: Approved for the treatment of FM by the US FDA in 2009, milnacipran (Savella® sold/marketed by Forest Pharmaceuticals) inhibits norepinephrine and serotonin reuptake, i.e., it potentiates (increases the effect of) the neurotransmitters norepinephrine and serotonin, both of which decrease the experience of pain and elevate mood. Of course, other non-drug treatments (such as nutrients and dietary optimization) can have the same effect, but most medical doctors have no training in nondrug treatments[37,38,39,40] and thus habitually turn to drugs as the one-and-only answer to the patients' problems[41], especially when these are sanctified by FDA/government approval. Nondrug treatments that enhance serotonergic

---

Black box warning for milnacipran/Savella

"Savella is a selective serotonin and norepinephrine reuptake inhibitor (SNRI), similar to some drugs used for the treatment of depression and other psychiatric disorders. Antidepressants increased the risk compared to placebo of suicidal thinking and behavior (suicidality) in children, adolescents, and young adults in short-term studies of major depressive disorder (MDD) and other psychiatric disorders."

http://www.frx.com/pi/Savella_pi.pdf, linked as "Full Prescribing Information" from http://www.savella.com/important-risk-information.aspx Accessed April 2012

---

and noradrenergic neurotransmission include exercise, relaxation, massage, and nutritional supplementation with omega-3 fatty acids (as found in fish oil), nutritional supplementation in general and vitamin D supplementation in particular. Adverse effects associated with use of milnacipran include seizures, suicidality, depression, worsening hypomania/mania, Stevens-Johnson syndrome (which is a medical emergency that can be fatal), serotonin syndrome, neuroleptic malignant syndrome, hypertensive (elevated blood pressure) crisis, tachycardia (rapid heart rate), hyponatremia (low sodium in the blood, which can occasionally result in permanent brain damage), abnormal bleeding (due to abnormal platelet function), glaucoma, and liver toxicity.[42] Treatment of fibromyalgia is the only FDA-approved use of this medication, which when used at the recommended dose of 50 mg twice daily costs $144 per month (pricing in April 2012). This drug is accompanied by a "black box warning" alerting physicians and patients to an increase in risk of suicide.

o **Cyclobenzaprine, Tramadol, and acetaminophen**: Cyclobenzaprine (a muscle-relaxing drug), Tramadol (a non-typical opioid, centrally-acting narcotic analgesic) and acetaminophen (centrally acting analgesic), show low efficacy and have little research supporting their use in the treatment of FM; these drugs also carry important risks for adverse effects, and they do not favorably alter the course of the disease over the long-term.[43] Per recent information from the American College of Rheumatology (ACR), treatment of FM with opioid drugs "may cause greater pain sensitivity or make pain persist."[44]

o **Exercise**: Low-intensity aerobic exercise may initially exacerbate symptoms but can result in very modest mental and physical improvement. Exercise alone cannot cure FM.

o **Cognitive-behavioral therapy (CBT)**: Cognitive-behavioral therapy helps patients deal with and adapt to the impact of the illness. Therapy alone cannot cure FM.

o **Patient (mis)education in standard medicine**: "Patient education" from a *medical* perspective generally means telling patients that ❶ they will probably have the condition forever, ❷ they will not immediately die from it, ❸ they need to take it seriously (i.e., comply with medical treatment), and ❹ they need to rely on drugs for alleviation of symptoms since no cause of the condition is known and therefore no direct treatment is available. From the medial perspective, these communications are considered "helpful" and "reassuring"; however, part of the effect that is created is **dependency** ("You need these drugs from me."), **passivity** ("There's nothing you can do about this, so don't even try to think for yourself or seek 'alternative' treatments."), and **co-victimization** ("We are both victims of our ignorance; I am in this with you in that we are both blind and dependent on drug management."). In the examples that follow, I will review and summarize patient educational materials from major medical journals; for efficiency, I will use quotes followed by my comments in *italics*:

- Patient education from American Academy of Family Physicians accessed April 2012 from the website FamilyDoctor.org[45]:
  - "your muscles and organs are not being damaged." — *This is false/inaccurate information. Several primary research studies have demonstrated consistently pathologic and biochemical abnormalities in muscle tissue from patients with fibromyalgia; this research has been published in widely available peer-reviewed medical journals.*
  - "This condition is not life-threatening, but it is chronic (ongoing). Although there is no cure,…" — *This is false information (the condition is curable); the statement as it reads produces patient passivity and drug-dependency, which is exactly what the medical profession and the drug industry wants.*
  - "There isn't currently a cure for fibromyalgia. Your care will focus on helping you minimize the impact of fibromyalgia on your life and treating your symptoms. Your doctor can prescribe medicine to help with your pain,… The treatment recommendations your doctor makes won't do any good unless you follow them." — *Again, false information that promotes passivity and medical-drug dependency.*
  - Weak recommendations under the guise of "taking an active role in your healthcare" include 1) maintaining a healthy outlook, 2) support groups, 3) **take medicines exactly as prescribed**, 4) moderate exercise, 5) stress management, 6) "establish healthy sleep habits", 7) make a routine daily schedule, 8) "make healthy lifestyle choices." *Most of these recommendations are blatantly passive, vague, and ineffective while fostering drug-dependency.*
- "Patient Education—Fibromyalgia" from the American College of Rheumatology accessed in April 2012 from the website Rheumatology.org[46]:
  - "Though there is no cure, medications can relieve symptoms." — *This is a commonly used statement within the medical community from doctors to patients to create passivity and drug/medical dependency.*
  - "There likely are certain genes that can make people more prone to getting fibromyalgia and the other health problems that can occur with it. Genes alone, though, do not cause fibromyalgia." — *These are common statements in the medical community, basically summed as "We don't know what we are doing but your only hope is to depend on us."*
  - "For the person with fibromyalgia, it is as though the "volume control" is turned up too high in the brain's pain processing centers." — *This promotes the concept of "primary central sensitization" (i.e., the brain has defied normal physiology and has somehow [without known cause, by itself] become too sensitive to pain); this "blame the brain" concept is used to leverage drug sales for pain-relieving and anti-depressant drugs as I have recently reviewed in video:* www.youtube.com/watch?v=41opevN87qs

- "There is no cure for fibromyalgia. However, symptoms can be treated with both medication and non-drug treatments." — *This is the standard "party line" for the medical profession, whose chief goal is not to cure diseases but rather to drug them indefinitely, thereby creating a perpetual audience for their services and prescriptions. Honorable mention (more accurately: dishonorable mention) is generally given to "lifestyle modification" but is generally done so in a way that provides vague advice for ineffective interventions, thereby* **creating the illusion of options** *while undercutting any potential for these "options" to actually work.*
- Non-drug treatments reviewed: relaxation, deep breathing, meditation, sleep, avoidance of nicotine and caffeine, exercise including such revelations as "take the stairs instead of the elevator, or park further [*sic*] away from the store", and "education" from other medical and special interest groups. *These are all essentially worthless suggestions, but they are effective distractions for patients and doctors so that effective treatments are marginalized and drug/medical dependency is fostered.*
- Prescription drugs are given the primary emphasis in the treatment section. *Whether drugs are effective or not, the medical profession relies on drugs for its position in society and will therefore advocate their use.*

The most common pattern in medical books and articles: components of the medical paradigm

1. Diseases are complex and incomprehensible: The condition generally is described as complex, with genetic factors, and of unknown cause.
2. Characteristics and diagnostic criteria are reviewed: The medical profession is very good at defining and diagnosing problems, but the reliance on drugs often detours from the more effective nondrug treatments.
3. Nondrug treatments are marginalized: Brief mention is made of diet and lifestyle and other non-drug treatments, but the information is nonspecific, very general, and almost always diluted to the point of inefficacy.
4. Authentic integrative and functional medicine approaches are essentially never mentioned: Generally, the only nondrug treatments that are mentioned are weak or are mentioned so casually that no action can be taken from the information presented.
5. Nearly always the disease is described as chronic and incurable: Even if a cure is known and published in available peer-reviewed research, most medical books and articles conclude that the causes are unknown and that drug treatment is warranted.
6. Drug treatments are emphasized: Drug benefits inflated and their adverse effects are minimized if mentioned at all.
7. Hope for the future is always placed back in the hands of "more research" and "drug development": Often some mention of "hope for the future" is made, generally in the guise of research and drug development; all the while, safe and effective non-drug treatment approaches that go far beyond diet and lifestyle are virtually never mentioned.

Functional Medicine Considerations, Assessments, and Interventions

- **Functional Medicine (FxMed) perspectives**: Two fundamental premises of Functional Medicine are: (1) chronic *diseases* are manifestations of chronic *dysfunctions*, and (2) dysfunction can result from a wide range of interconnected genotropic (gene-influenced), metabolic, nutritional, microbial, inflammatory, toxic, environmental, and psychological and social influences. **Many of these dysfunctions lie outside the narrow, pathology-based, pharmacocentric (drug-centered) view of standard allopathic medicine**. The functional medicine approach to each individual fibromyalgia patient is based on the presumption that the condition has an underlying primary cause (or several interconnected causes) and that the cause(s) can be identified and addressed. The cause(s) may be manifold and multifaceted and may differ among patients with the same diagnostic label. The FxMed approach includes the diagnostic and therapeutic considerations of standard medicine but extends far beyond these in assessment, treatment, and understanding. Clinicians trained in FxMed appreciate that as a diagnostic label, fibromyalgia is commonly applied to any patient with chronic, widespread pain and that the current trend to limit diagnostic evaluation in such patients will clearly result in failure to identify and address readily diagnosable and treatable problems that can result in a clinical picture that resembles FM. Clinicians must consider chronic infections (such as with hepatitis C virus, *Borrelia burgdorferi* [the bacteria strongly associated with Lyme disease], *Chlamydia/Chlamydophila pneumoniae*, and the protozoan parasite *Babesia*, which is also associated with Lyme disease and co-infection with *Borrelia burgdorferi*), cancerous conditions such as multiple myeloma and lymphoma, and autoimmune/rheumatic diseases such as polymyositis and polymyalgia rheumatica. A few of the other more exemplary conditions to consider in patients with widespread pain are vitamin D deficiency, hypothyroidism, iron overload, and chronic exposure to and accumulation of xenobiotics—perhaps most importantly mercury and lead.

  The Functional Medicine Matrix, which is copyrighted and periodically updated by Institute for Functional Medicine (IFM, http://www.functionalmedicine.org/) is a graphic representation of the interconnected and interdependent nature of the major organ systems and physiologic processes. The diagram is used as a teaching tool for doctors to help them appreciate major concepts in Functional Medicine, and it also serves as a teaching tool for patients who likewise benefit from appreciating that the body functions as a whole, with each major system affecting the others.

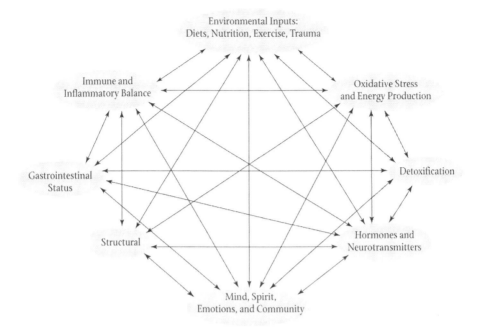

The Functional Medicine Matrix circa 2003-2006 diagrammed by Vasquez for the Institute for Functional Medicine (IFM): The "Matrix" has been used as a teaching tool for doctors and an educational tool for patients to apprehend the interconnected and interdependent nature of various organ systems and physiologic processes in the genesis of health and disease. Reproduced here as published in Vasquez A. Web-like Interconnections of Physiological Factors. *Integrative Medicine: A Clinician's Journal* 2006, April/May, 32-37. The Functional Medicine Matrix and has been updated by IFM (FunctionalMedicine.org) several times since this model was originally diagrammed by Dr Vasquez.

Conditions that Mimic (or Contribute to) the Clinical of Fibromyalgia

- **Vitamin D deficiency**: A clinical picture nearly identical to fibromyalgia— chronic widespread pain, mental depression/anxiety, headaches, low-grade systemic inflammation—can result from vitamin D deficiency.[47] Fibromyalgia patients are commonly deficient in vitamin D, and indeed, **vitamin D deficiency—with its attendant pain, anxiety/depression, and normal lab values on routine laboratory testing—is often misdiagnosed as fibromyalgia**, as reported by Holick.[48] Increased severity of the deficiency correlates with worsening depression and anxiety in these patients.[49] Correction of vitamin D deficiency by administration of vitamin D3 (cholecalciferol) in doses of 5,000-10,000 IU (international units) per day for several months has resulted in a dramatic alleviation of pain; such intervention among patients with low back pain has resulted in cure rates greater than 95%.[50] Other studies with vitamin D3 using doses 400-4,000 IU/day have shown that vitamin D3 supplementation for the correction of vitamin D deficiency alleviates depression and enhances sense of well-being. Vitamin D3 supplementation—or adequate endogenous production from ultraviolet light exposure (approximately 10-30 minutes per day of full-body exposure at midday, near the equator)—to meet physiological requirements of approximately 4,000 IU/day is safe and results in numerous major health benefits.[51,52,53] The only risk associated with vitamin D supplementation is hypercalcemia—too much calcium in the blood, mostly as a result of increased gastrointestinal absorption of calcium; hypercalcemia can cause abdominal pain, bone pain, fatigue, constipation, abnormal heart rhythm (arrhythmia), kidney stones, increased thirst and urination [additional details[54]]. Hypercalcemia caused solely by vitamin D3 supplementation is extremely rare; vitamin D supplementation in the range of 2,000 – 10,000 IU per day for adults is remarkably safe.[55,56] The main drug-nutrient interaction of relevance to vitamin D supplementation is with the drug hydrochlorothiazide, which is a diuretic drug used for the treatment of high blood pressure; this drug causes calcium retention by the kidney and when combined with vitamin D supplementation may lead to high levels of calcium in the blood (hypercalcemia). *Note from Dr Vasquez: I have only seen this occur one time in my clinical practice in a hypertensive patient taking hydrochlorothiazide who was vitamin D deficient; vitamin D supplementation at 2,000 IU/d caused a mild hypercalcemia within 10 days which was treated simply by discontinuing the vitamin D supplementation (also note that discontinuation of appropriate nutritional supplementation in favor of continuing a symptom-suppressing drug is generally not my preference but in this particular situation it was the best choice).* A group of conditions called granulomatous diseases—which can include lymphoma, sarcoidosis, and Crohn's disease—increase the risk for hypercalcemia; caution and more frequent laboratory monitoring must be employed when using physiological doses of vitamin D3 in patients with these conditions. Diagnosis of vitamin D3 deficiency is simple and is based upon measurement of serum 25-hydroxy vitamin D3 (25[OH]D) levels. Supplementation effectiveness and safety are monitored by measuring 25(OH)D levels and serum calcium, respectively. The two goals with supplementation of vitamin D3 are ❶ safety—avoidance of hypercalcemia or any calcium-related complications, and ❷ efficacy—serum 25[OH]D levels should enter into the optimal range of 50 – 100 ng/mL (125 - 250 nmol/L) per Vasquez[57,58] and Vasquez et al[59,60,61] as demonstrated in the illustration.

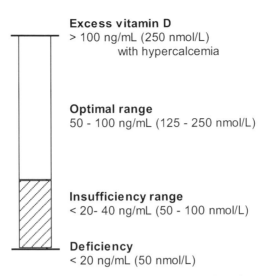

Excess vitamin D
> 100 ng/mL (250 nmol/L)
with hypercalcemia

Optimal range
50 - 100 ng/mL (125 - 250 nmol/L)

Insufficiency range
< 20- 40 ng/mL (50 - 100 nmol/L)

Deficiency
< 20 ng/mL (50 nmol/L)

Interpretation of serum 25(OH) vitamin D levels. Modified from Vasquez et al, *Alternative Therapies in Health and Medicine* 2004. Vasquez A. *Musculoskeletal Pain: Expanded Clinical Strategies* (Institute for Functional Medicine) 2008. Vasquez A. *Nutritional Perspectives* 2011 January

- **Functional/metabolic hypothyroidism**: Insufficient levels of thyroid hormone lead to an associated clinical condition called hypothyroidism (*hypo*=low, *thyroidism*=thyroid condition). Both mild and overt hypothyroidism are well known in the rheumatology literature as causes of diffuse body pain. As a cause of diffuse muscle pain, mild-moderate hypothyroidism can mimic fibromyalgia; more severe cases of hypothyroidism cause "hypothyroid myopathy" which typically manifests as polymyositis-like disease with proximal muscle weakness and an increased blood level of the enzyme creatine kinase, indicating muscle damage. In its most extreme, hypothyroid myopathy presents as muscle enlargement (pseudohypertrophy); in adults, this condition is called Hoffmann syndrome while in children it is known as Kocher-Debré-Sémélaigne syndrome.[62] Hypothyroidism is well known to cause depression and low-grade systemic inflammation; these are two findings common in FM. Another related problem commonly seen with both FM and hypothyroidism is IBS and small intestinal bacterial overgrowth (SIBO); hypothyroidism causes a slowing of intestinal motility, promoting stasis in the gastrointestinal tract which leads to an overgrowth of bacteria.[63] Detailed thyroid assessment should include measurements of thyroid stimulating hormone (TSH), free T4, free T3, total T3, reverse T3 (rT3), and antithyroid peroxidase (anti-TPO) and antithyroglobulin antibodies. *Note from Dr Vasquez: A very comprehensive overview of the diagnosis and treatment of hypothyroidism in its various forms—primary, secondary, and a form of hypothyroidism caused by impaired conversion of the inactive T4 hormone to the active T3 hormone (referred to as metabolic or peripheral hypothyroidism)—is detailed in my book <u>Migraine Headaches, Hypothyroidism, and Fibromyalgia</u> published in 2012; treatment with active thyroid hormone—T3—and nutritional and dietary interventions are emphasized.*

Terminology related to thyroid hormone production and metabolism

- <u>TSH—thyroid stimulating hormone</u>: Hormone secreted from the anterior pituitary gland to stimulate T4 and T3 production from the thyroid gland.
- <u>T4</u>: The inactive form of thyroid hormone, accounting for about 80% of thyroid gland output.
- <u>T3</u>: The active form of thyroid hormone produced from conversion of T4, accounts for about 20% of thyroid gland output. This is the form of thyroid hormone that is most important, because it is active and ready to stimulate metabolic processes.
- <u>rT3—reverse T3</u>: During times of stress and also as a result of some drugs, T4 is preferentially converted to rT3, which is inactive and may actually impair the utilization of active T3. In some people, especially after a period of severe emotional stress, their thyroid hormone metabolism becomes skewed toward rT3 production, perhaps as an adaptive mechanism to conserve energy. However, increased rT3 production results in impaired thyroid hormone function and thereby promotes a clinical picture of hypothyroidism (low function of the thyroid gland) even when gland function is adequate; the problem is the hormone's peripheral metabolism, not its production from the gland.

```
FREE T3/REVERSE T3 RATIO
  FREE T3/REVERSE T3 RATIO                        0.93 L        1.05-1.91**
  FREE T3                          325                          230-420 pg/dL
  REVERSE T3                                       350 H        100-340*** pg/mL
      **Ratio= Free T3 in pg/dL : reverse T3 in pg/mL. Ratio for reference
      range is calculated by dividing the lower and upper end of free T3
      with the mean of reverse T3 (220 pg/mL).

      ***Observed reference range is reported for reverse T3 per client
      request.

      This test was performed using a kit that has not been approved or
      cleared by the FDA. The analytical performance characteristics of this
      test have been determined by Quest Diagnostics Nichols Institute, San
      Juan Capistrano. This test should not be used for diagnosis without
      confirmation by other medically established means.
```

A 42yo male with fatigue and elevated rT3 levels indicating functional hypothyroidism

: This is an example of a case of functional/metabolic hypothyroidism, which is due to impaired peripheral conversion of inactive thyroxine (T4) into its active form triiodothyronine (T3) and an excess production of reverse T3 (rT3). Patients with this condition typically benefit from receiving prescription T3 rather than the more commonly used T4; the goal is to temporarily suppress endogenous T4 production so that enzymes in the converting pathway are temporarily downregulated and thus peripheral thyroid metabolism has an opportunity to recalibrate and remain normal following the withdrawal of thyroid hormone supplementation.[64,65]

Date and Time Collected	Date Entered	Date and Time Reported	Physician Name	NPI	Ph
02/04/10 11:41	02/04/10	02/09/10 04:06ET			19(

Tests Ordered

Triiodothyronine (T3);Reverse T3;Triiodothyronine,Free,Serum

General Comments

PID: 8282293

TESTS	RESULT	FLAG	UNITS	REFERENCE INTERV
Triiodothyronine (T3)				
Triiodothyronine (T3)	57	Low	ng/dL	71-180
Reverse T3				
Reverse T3	312		pg/mL	90-350
Triiodothyronine,Free,Serum				
Triiodothyronine,Free,Serum	2.5		pg/mL	2.0-4.4

A 38yo male with fatigue and depressed T3 levels indicating functional hypothyroidism

: This is an example of a case of functional/metabolic hypothyroidism, which is due to impaired peripheral conversion of inactive thyroxine (T4) into its active form triiodothyronine (T3) and an excess production of reverse T3 (rT3). Patients with this condition typically benefit from receiving prescription T3 rather than the more commonly used T4; the goal is to temporarily suppress endogenous T4 production so that enzymes in the converting pathway are temporarily downregulated and thus peripheral thyroid metabolism has an opportunity to recalibrate and remain normal following the withdrawal of thyroid hormone supplementation.[66,67]

- <u>Occult infections, especially with *Mycoplasma* species and *Chlamydia/Chlamydophila* pneumoniae</u>: Clinicians are increasingly appreciating the role of occult intracellular infections in the genesis and/or perpetuation of chronic health problems, including some previously perplexing problems such as chronic fatigue syndrome (CFS), inflammatory arthritis, and multiple sclerosis (MS). For chronic *Chlamydophila* (previously *Chlamydia*) *pneumoniae* infection, testing for serum levels of antibodies is useful followed by treatment with antibacterial drugs such as azithromycin and nutritional supplements such as N-acetyl-cysteine (NAC) in appropriately selected patients; for chronic *Mycoplasma* infections, because of the various subspecies involved, polymerase chain reaction (PCR) testing appears to be preferred followed by treatment with doxycycline in adults.

  o <u>Clinical investigation: Prevalence of antibodies to *Chlamydophila* pneumoniae in persons without clinical evidence of respiratory infection (*Journal of Clinical Pathology* 2002 May[68])</u>: The authors note that "Because there is as yet no standardization of serological criteria for persistent infection, we considered antibody titers of > 1/20 in the IgA fraction, together with **IgG titers of 1/64 to 1/256, to be indicative of persistent infection.**" This article supports clinical experience and post-graduate presentations[69] showing that in persons with fatigue and various other chronic health disorders characterized by pain and inflammation (such as chronic inflammatory arthritis[70] or spine[71] inflammation), the finding of IgG antibody levels >1:64 suggests that the patient has a persistent *Chlamydophila pneumoniae* infection which may be alleviated by the administration of—for example—the antibiotic **azithromycin** (adult dose 250 mg every other day due to the drug's long half-life, given for several weeks or months until symptoms are resolved and/or antibody titers are normalized) and **N-acetyl-cysteine** (NAC: 500-1,200 mg 1-3 times per day by mouth between meals). Positive antibody titers (levels) are common because the infection itself is common *as a transient condition*; the issue here is the determination of which patients have a *chronic* and *persistent* low-grade infection. The finding of an elevated antibody titer—that is a level greater than 1:64—indicates the need to consider long-term antimicrobial intervention. A brief case report from the author's experience is provided below:

```
Chlamydia pneumoniae IgG      >1:256    High       08/29/11
Chlamydia pneumoniae IgM       <1:10               Neg:<1:16
                                                   Neg:<1:10
```

Elevated titers to *Chlamydia/Chlamydophila pneumoniae* suggesting chronic persistent infection in a 40yo male physician *without pulmonary symptoms* but with a positive history of chronic sinus congestion and low-grade fatigue— improvement with azithromycin and NAC: This patient experienced years of severe psychologic and physiologic stress during medical school to then have an acute upper respiratory illness onset in September 2010 while working in a Family Medicine residency program; recurrent bouts of upper respiratory illness—attributed to viral infections—persisted for five months until February 2011. By the summer of 2011, the patient was relatively asymptomatic except for persistent sinus congestion and low-grade fatigue. No pulmonary symptoms such as shortness of breath were ever present. Following detection of the elevated antibody titer, the patient started on azithromycin and NAC as described above, which resulted in a short-term (12-hour) exacerbation of symptoms followed by complete and sustained resolution of sinus congestion and improved energy levels and exercise endurance.[72]

- o Review: *Mycoplasma* blood infection in chronic fatigue and fibromyalgia syndromes (*Rheumatology International* 2003 Sep[73]): The author notes that "**Chronic fatigue syndrome (CFS) and fibromyalgia syndrome (FMS)** are characterized by a lack of consistent laboratory and clinical abnormalities. Although they are distinguishable as separate syndromes based on established criteria, a great number of patients are diagnosed with both." He goes on to say, "In studies using **polymerase chain reaction [PCR] methods**, **mycoplasma blood infection has been detected in about 50% of patients with CFS and/or FMS**, including patients with Gulf War illnesses and symptoms that overlap with one or both syndromes. **Such infection is detected in only about 10% of healthy individuals**, significantly less than in patients. Most patients with CFS/FMS who have mycoplasma infection appear to recover and reach their pre-illness state after **long-term antibiotic therapy with doxycycline**, and the infection cannot be detected after recovery. … It is not clear whether mycoplasmas are associated with CFS/FMS as causal agents, cofactors, or opportunistic infections in patients with immune disturbances. Whether mycoplasma infection can be detected in about 50% of all patient populations with CFS and/or FMS is yet to be determined."

- o Clinical investigation: High prevalence of Mycoplasmal infections in symptomatic (chronic fatigue syndrome) family members of *Mycoplasma*-positive Gulf War illness patients (*Journal of Chronic Fatigue Syndrome* 2003[74]): The authors state, "…a relatively common finding in Gulf War Illness patients is a bacterial infection due to *Mycoplasma* species, we examined military families (149 patients: 42 veterans, 40 spouses, 32 other relatives and 35 children with at least one family complaint of illness) selected from a **group of 110 veterans with Gulf War Illness who tested positive (~41%) for at least one of four** *Mycoplasma* **species**: *M. fermentans, M. hominis, M. pneumoniae* or *M. genitalium.* Consistent with previous results, over 80% of Gulf War Illness patients who were positive for blood mycoplasmal infections had **only one** *Mycoplasma* **species, in particular** *M. fermentans* (Odds ratio = 17.9, P <0.001). In healthy control subjects the incidence of mycoplasmal infection was ~8.5% and none were found to have multiple mycoplasmal species."

- **Hemochromatosis and iron overload**: Genetic hemochromatosis is a common iron-accumulation disease that causes chronic persistent musculoskeletal pain, even while most routine laboratory tests are normal; thus, the clinical presentation of iron overload may be confused with that of fibromyalgia. Hemochromatosis is one of the most common hereditary disorders among Caucasians, with a homozygote (two of the same genes, results in more severe disease) frequency of approximately 1 in 200 to 250 persons and a heterozygote (only one affected gene, less severe disease) frequency of approximately 1 in 7 persons. Various other hereditary iron overload disorders affect all races, with the highest prevalence in persons of African descent (as high as 1 in 80 according to some small studies among hospitalized African-American patients).[75,76] Eighty percent of hemochromatosis patients have chronic musculoskeletal pain, which is commonly the earliest or only presenting complaint.[77] In contrast to the clinical presentation of FM, the musculoskeletal manifestations of iron overload are classically arthritic (i.e., in the joints) rather than muscular, with the joints of the hands, wrists, hips, and knees most commonly affected. However, due to the widespread distribution of pain and the normalcy of routine laboratory results, iron overload can mimic fibromyalgia. Given the high population prevalence of iron overload and the high frequency with which it presents with musculoskeletal manifestations, **all patients with chronic, nontraumatic musculoskeletal pain must be tested for iron overload.** Serum ferritin, which can be used alone or with transferrin saturation, is the best single laboratory test; confirmed results greater than 200 mcg/L in women and 300 mcg/L in men necessitate treatment with diagnostic and therapeutic phlebotomy (therapeutic "blood donation" is the most effective treatment for chronic iron overload).[78] *Note from Dr Vasquez: Additional details about the etiologies, diagnosis, and comprehensive treatment of iron overload are available at my website: http://OptimalHealthResearch.com/hemochromatosis.html*

- **Accumulation of xenobiotics (including mercury and lead):** Xenobiotic (foreign chemical) accumulation may occasionally cause widespread pain resembling fibromyalgia, and xenobiotic detoxification (depuration) can alleviate pain in affected patients. Toxic chemical and toxic metal accumulation is common in humans worldwide and has been well-documented in Americans. Eight percent (8%) of American women of childbearing age have sufficiently high levels of mercury in their blood to increase the risk of health problems such as neurological damage in their children.[79] Americans in general show alarmingly high concentrations and combinations of neurotoxic (nerve-damaging), carcinogenic (cancer-causing), diabetogenic (diabetes-causing), and immunotoxic (immune-altering) xenobiotics/toxins.[80] Adverse effects of toxic chemicals (e.g., pesticides, herbicides, solvents, plastics, formaldehyde, petroleum byproducts) and heavy metals (especially lead and mercury) are well described throughout the biomedical literature and have been clinically reviewed by Crinnion.[81,82,83,84] Among toxins with the ability to produce chronic muscle pain, mercury may deserve special recognition given its ubiquitous distribution in the human population and the scientific evidence detailing its numerous adverse effects.[85,86] Whether by metabolic, neurological, or endocrinologic means, occult mercury toxicity may manifest as a syndrome of widespread muscle pain that resembles fibromyalgia.[87] Acrodynia is a subacute peripheral pain syndrome due to mercury toxicity classically seen in children.[88] Acute mercury intoxication can result in severe skeletal muscle damage (rhabdomyolysis).[89] Mercury in organic and inorganic forms interferes with acetylcholine

---

Potential benefits of reducing the body burden of mercury in patients with chronic pain and fatigue

"We suggest that **metal-driven inflammation** may affect the hypothalamic-pituitary-adrenal axis (HPA axis) and indirectly trigger psychosomatic multisymptoms characterizing **chronic fatigue syndrome, fibromyalgia**, and other diseases of unknown etiology."

Sterzl I, et al. Mercury and nickel allergy: risk factors in fatigue and autoimmunity. *Neuro Endocrinol Lett.* 1999;20(3-4):221-228

---

reception and several crucial aspects of the sarcoplasmic reticulum, including calcium-magnesium-ATPase and calcium transport; these adverse effects establish a molecular basis for a *mercurial myopathy* (mercury-induced muscle disease).[90,91] The toxicity of mercury is greatly increased by simultaneous accumulation of lead, elevated levels of which are also common in the U.S. population. Demonstration of high mercury and lead levels in urine following administration of a chelating agent such as dimercaptosuccinic acid (DMSA) can be used to diagnose chronic mercury or lead overload, and orally administered DMSA is also used for treatment.[92,93,94,95] Failure to preadminister a chelating agent prior to measurement of urine mercury renders the test insensitive for chronic accumulation and can thus give the false impression that mercury is not contributory to fibromyalgia, as concluded by Kotter et al.[96] Orally administered selenium, phytochelatins (metal-binding peptides from plants[97]), a high-fiber diet, and potassium citrate can be used to augment mercury excretion.[98]

- o Clinical investigation: Reduced exposure to xenobiotics (cosmetics) alleviates fibromyalgia (*Journal of Women's Health* 2004 Mar[99]): Women tend to use more cosmetics than men, and—given that cosmetic products are foreign chemicals with potentially adverse effects—this study was conducted to determine if avoidance of cosmetics would alleviate symptoms of FM. The author of this report describes a prospective, randomized, controlled trial of 48 women with FM (some of whom had a rheumatic condition) who were regular users of cosmetics was carried out to investigate if a reduced use of cosmetics would reduce the symptoms. The patients were told to avoid or completely abstain from using all ointments, creams, skin lotions, pain-relieving liniments, cleaning lotions, oil treatments, hair-coloring chemicals, and tanning lotion; they were also advised to reduce their use of soap and shampoo, both of which—like skin creams—are generally formulated with perfumes and other chemicals and applied to large regions of the body. This research showed that, after 2 years, FM patients who reduced their exposure to chemicals/xenobiotics/cosmetics experienced significant reductions in pain, sleep disturbances, and musculoskeletal stiffness ($p < 0.02$), together with better physical function and improved sense of well-being as measured by the Fibromyalgia Impact Questionnaire (FIQ). Thus, avoiding chemical exposure appears to provide no-cost no-risk therapeutic benefit to FM patients by alleviating pain and improving several indicators of overall health.

- o Case report: Therapeutic detoxification to reduce the body burden of toxic metals (lead and mercury) in a woman diagnosed with FM leads to complete relief of FM symptoms: This 54-year-old athletic female with healthy diet, lifestyle, and supportive relationship presented with chronic diffuse musculoskeletal pain. Health history was significant for decades of environmental illness/intolerance (EI) also known as multiple chemical sensitivity (MCS). Family history was positive for maternal temporal (giant cell) arteritis, an autoimmune disease characterized by inflamed arteries in the neck, head, and shoulders. Physical examination revealed numerous tender points consistent with fibromyalgia. The patient's history and stool analysis (comprehensive bacteriology and parasitology, tests for intestinal "infections") were unremarkable and unsupportive of either identifiable infection or nonspecific bacterial overgrowth. Laboratory investigations revealed normal results for hsCRP (high-sensitity c-reactive protein, a marker for inflammation), CK (creatine kinase, a marker of muscle damage and myositis), ANA (anti-nuclear antibodies, elevated in many autoimmune diseases such as lupus/SLE), vitamin D, calcium, phosphorus, and comprehensive thyroid evaluation. The patient was then (defensively) referred to an excellent osteopathic medical internist who diagnosed the patient with fibromyalgia. The patient was unsatisfied with the diagnosis of FM and returned to the current author, who then performed urine heavy metal testing provoked with 10 mg per kilogram of dimercaptosuccinic acid (DMSA). Results revealed the highest levels of lead and mercury encountered in the author's practice at that time. As in the accompanying lab results, lead levels were 6x above the reference range and mercury levels were 7x above the reference range. The patient was commenced on DMSA 10 mg/kg/d three days "on" and 4 days "off" (cyclic dosing is used to avoid toxicity in general and bone marrow toxicity [neutropenia] in particular), selenium 800 mcg/d to promote excretion of toxic metals and to support renal and antioxidant protection, vegetable juices to provide potassium and citrate for urinary alkalinization and enhanced excretion of xenobiotics[100], and a proprietary phytochelatin (metal-binding peptides from plants) concentrate to bind toxic metals in the gut and thereby promote their fecal excretion by blocking enterohepatic recycling/recirculation. DMSA chelation is approved by the US Food and Drug Administration (FDA) for the treatment of lead toxicity in children.[101] The use of DMSA for children and adults is supported by peer-reviewed literature[102,103,104,105,106] and has been reviewed in more detail by this author in *Integrative Rheumatology*[107] and to a lesser extent in the peer-reviewed monograph for continuing medical education (CME) *Musculoskeletal Pain: Expanded Clinical Strategies*.[108] After approximately 8 months of treatment, the patient was completely free of pain, and the clinical improvement was associated with a reduction in both lead and mercury of approximately 50% as demonstrated by follow-up laboratory testing. This case was published in peer-reviewed literature for continuing education credits for physicians.[109]

				Date Completed:	10/22/2005
Lead	30	<	5		
Mercury	21	<	3		

				Date Completed:	6/30/2006
Lead	15	<	5		
Mercury	8.2	<	4		

Marked accumulation of lead and mercury in a patient diagnosed with FM—complete elimination of pain and stiffness following identification and reduction in the body burden of lead and mercury: *Presentation*: 54yo woman presents with nontraumatic widespread pain consistent with a diagnosis of fibromyalgia; the diagnosis of FM is confirmed by two clinicians. All laboratory test results were normal except for urine toxic metal testing which showed 6x elevations of lead and 7x elevations of mercury. Treatment for lead and mercury toxicity was started as described above and the patient experienced safe and effective alleviation of all pain after 8 months of treatment; reductions in pain correlated directly with reductions in body burden of lead and mercury.

Small intestine bacterial overgrowth (SIBO) is the ultimate cause of and most logical explanation for FM:

- Small intestine bacterial overgrowth (SIBO)—also referred to as "intestinal bacterial overgrowth" or simply "bacterial overgrowth"—provides the single best model for explaining the clinical and pathophysiological manifestations of fibromyalgia. Although commonly underappreciated by many clinicians, SIBO is common in clinical practice, affecting for example approximately 40% of patients with rheumatoid arthritis, 84% of patients with IBS, and 90% to 100% of patients with fibromyalgia. **In a study of 42 fibromyalgia patients, all 42 FM patients showed laboratory evidence of SIBO, and the severity of the intestinal bacterial overgrowth correlated positively with the severity of the fibromyalgia**, thus indicating the plausibility of a causal relationship.[110] The links between fibromyalgia and IBS are also strong; **most IBS patients meet strict diagnostic criteria for fibromyalgia, and most fibromyalgia patients meet strict criteria for IBS**. Lubrano et al[111] showed that fibromyalgia severity correlated with IBS severity among patients who met strict diagnostic criteria for both conditions. The high degree of overlap between these two diagnostic labels suggests that these conditions are two variations of a common pathophysiological process—SIBO.[112] SIBO causes altered bowel function, immune activation, and visceral hypersensitivity, and it is the best causative explanation for the clinical and pathophysiological manifestations of IBS; for more details and citations, see the excellent review by Lin published in *Journal of the American Medical Association* in 2004.[113] IBS is characterized by *visceral* hyperalgesia (hypersensitivity to pain), just as fibromyalgia is characterized by *skeletal muscle* hyperalgesia. Given that strong evidence indicates that IBS is caused by SIBO and that IBS and fibromyalgia are variations of the same pathophysiological process, then fibromyalgia may therefore be caused by SIBO. However, these links and interconnections require substantiation, as provided below.

A practical summary of SIBO: small intestine bacterial overgrowth
1. Definition: Generalized nonspecific overpopulation of bacteria (commonly with other microbes such as yeast) in the small intestine (and large intestine, too).
2. Frequency: Very common in clinical practice and the general population.
3. Primary symptoms: Gas and bloating, especially after carbohydrate consumption; may also have constipation and/or diarrhea.
4. Secondary symptoms: Fatigue, muscle aches, difficulty with concentration and cognition ("brain fog"), nutritional deficiencies due to malabsorption, immune activation due to absorption of microbial debris and metabolites.
5. Diagnosis: ❶ Based on the symptoms above, ❷ jejunal aspiration is the gold standard but is expensive, cumbersome, and potentially hazardous, ❸ measurement of fermentation products (hydrogen and methane) in breath following consumption of a carbohydrate such as glucose, sucrose, or lactulose; the amount of "gas" produced is proportional to the bacterial population, ❹ may find elevated short chain fatty acids (SCFA) in stool or elevated folate in blood, but not all cases of SIBO produce SCFA or folate, ❺ clinical response to low-carbohydrate diet and/or antibiotic drugs or antimicrobial herbs. The current author (AV) uses #1 in conjunction with #5 most commonly.
6. Treatments: Low-carbohydrate diet with antibiotic drugs (e.g., rifamixin (200 or 550 mg each) 400-550 mg tid po [1,200-1,650 mg daily] for 10-30 days) or antimicrobial herbs (e.g., time-released emulsified oregano oil 600 mg daily for 4-6 weeks, and/or berberine 400-1,000 mg daily for 4 weeks).

- *What is the evidence linking fibromyalgia with SIBO? What are the molecular mechanisms by which absorbed toxins and metabolites from SIBO can contribute to muscle pain and the mitochondrial/ATP/energy defects and the muscle tissue abnormalities seen in fibromyalgia patients?*
    1. Small intestine bacterial overgrowth is highly prevalent in fibromyalgia: Several studies have shown that 90% to 100% of fibromyalgia patients have evidence of SIBO; such a strong correlation and the dose-response relationship imply causality and must be integrated into any science-based model of fibromyalgia.
        - Clinical study: Patients with FM have evidence of frequent and severe bacterial overgrowth in the intestines (*Annals of the Rheumatic Diseases* 2004 Apr[114]): The **breath hydrogen test** is used for the detection of SIBO and involves orally administering a carbohydrate (such as lactulose, a source of sugar for bacteria) which is converted to hydrogen through bacterial fermentation; the exhaled hydrogen in the breath is measured as an indirect quantification of the amount of bacteria in the intestines. In this study, 20% of "healthy" control patients were found to have intestinal bacterial overgrowth via an abnormal hydrogen breath test compared with 93/111 (84%) subjects with IBS and **42/42 (100%) with fibromyalgia**. Subjects with fibromyalgia had

higher hydrogen production (indicating more severe SIBO), peak hydrogen, and area under the curve than subjects with IBS. **The degree of somatic pain in fibromyalgia correlates significantly with the hydrogen level seen on the breath test**.

2. <u>Fibromyalgia is tightly correlated with irritable bowel syndrome, a condition caused by small intestine bacterial overgrowth</u>: Fibromyalgia and IBS are strongly convergent, and the evidence indicates that IBS is caused largely or completely by SIBO; again, for more details and citations, see the brilliant article by Lin, cited previously.

3. <u>Small intestine bacterial overgrowth leads to systemic absorption of toxins that impair brain/nerve and muscle/mitochondrial function</u>: SIBO is associated with overproduction and absorption of bacterial cellular debris (e.g., lipopolysaccharide [LPS], bacterial DNA, peptidoglycans, teichoic acid, exotoxins) and antimetabolites—substances which are directly toxic to cellular energy/ATP production and muscle and nerve function—such as D-lactic acid, tyramine, tartaric acid, hydrogen sulfide. Intestinal gram-negative bacteria produce endotoxin (also known as lipopolysaccharide, LPS), which impairs skeletal muscle energy/ATP production (by stimulating skeletal muscle sodium-potassium-ATPase). Endotoxin also raises blood lactate (indicating impaired cellular energy production) under aerobic conditions in humans.[115] **Thus, via direct and indirect effects on cellular metabolism, chronic low-dose bacterial LPS/endotoxin exposure can result in impaired muscle metabolism and reduced ATP synthesis via impairment of mitochondrial function.** Intestinal bacteria also produce D-lactate, a well-known metabolic toxin in humans; SIBO often results in variable levels of D-lactate acidosis, severe cases of which can progress from fatigue and malaise to encephalopathy (e.g., confusion, ataxia, slurred speech, altered mental status) and death.[116] Supporting the proposal that bacterial overgrowth with D-lactate-producing bacteria is a contributor to the chronic fatigue syndromes including fibromyalgia is an excellent study published in 2009 showing that **patients with chronic fatigue syndrome have intestinal overgrowth of bacteria that produce the cellular toxin D-lactate**; specifically the research showed that these chronic fatigue patients have **a 7-fold increase in D-lactate producing *Enterococcus* and 1,100-fold increase in D-lactate producing *Streptococcus*.** Energy/ATP underproduction

and lactate overproduction cause muscle fatigue and muscle pain. An additional cellular toxin produced by intestinal bacteria is hydrogen sulfide (H2S), which causes DNA damage[117] (noted previously to be increased in fibromyalgia patients) and which impairs cellular energy production, a finding relevant to *but not necessarily limited to* the pathogenesis of ulcerative colitis.[118,119] Bacteria and yeast in the intestines produce H2S, which can bind to the mitochondrial enzyme cytochrome c oxidase (part of Complex IV of the electron transport chain), thereby impairing oxidative phosphorylation and ATP production; this may partly explain the association of gastrointestinal dysbiosis and small intestine bacterial overgrowth (SIBO) with conditions such as chronic fatigue syndrome (CFS) and fibromyalgia.[120]

Mitophagy: Destruction of mitochondria
"The removal of damaged mitochondria that could contribute to cellular dysfunction or death is achieved through process of mitochondrial autophagy, i.e. mitophagy."*
"Mitochondrial number and health are regulated by mitophagy, a process by which excessive or damaged mitochondria are subjected to autophagic degradation."**
"Autophagy can be beneficial for the cells by eliminating dysfunctional mitochondria, but massive autophagy can promote cell injury and may contribute to the pathophysiology of FM (fibromyalgia)."*
*Novak I. *Antioxid Redox Signal*. 2011 **Rambold. *Cell Cycle*. 2011 ***Cordero. *Arthritis Res Ther*. 2010

- Experimental study: Effect of *E. coli* endotoxin on mitochondrial form and function. (*Annals of Surgery* 1971 Dec[121]): Authors of this paper show that treatment of normal rat liver mitochondria with *E. coli* endotoxin results in mitochondrial impairment. They note previous research showing that animal exposure to *E. coli* endotoxin causes inhibition of mitochondrial respiration and uncoupling of oxidative phosphorylation. Near their conclusion, the authors write, "Thus we have evidence to show that topical ***E. coli* endotoxin has pathologic effects on both membrane integrity and internal mechanochemical systems of isolated mitochondria**." Readers should appreciate that *E. coli* is a common inhabitant of the gastrointestinal tract of humans and that its population is quantitatively increased during states of bacterial overgrowth of the small bowel, as is commonly seen in most patients with fibromyalgia. More recently, research has shown that impairment of mitochondrial function (noted in patients with fibromyalgia) can lead to destruction of mitochondria by a process termed "mitophagy" (noted in patients with fibromyalgia); over time, loss of mitochondria via mitophagy leads to reduced numbers of mitochondria in muscle and other tissues (noted in patients with fibromyalgia) and contributes to the fatigue and other symptoms which characterize FM.

▫ Clinical study: Increased D-lactic acid intestinal bacteria in patients with chronic fatigue syndrome (*In Vivo* 2009 Jul-Aug[122]): This excellent clinical research fully supports the pathoetiologic (disease causation) model presented in this chapter, which is derived and updated from a previous publication by this author: Vasquez A. *Musculoskeletal Pain: Expanded Clinical Strategies* published by the Institute for Functional Medicine in 2008. The authors of this 2009 study state in the summary of their research, "Patients with chronic fatigue syndrome (CFS) are affected by symptoms of cognitive dysfunction and neurological impairment, the cause of which has yet to be elucidated. However, these symptoms are strikingly similar to those of patients presented with D-lactic acidosis. A significant increase of Gram-positive facultative anaerobic fecal microorganisms in 108 CFS patients as compared to 177 control subjects is presented in this report. The viable count of D-lactic acid producing *Enterococcus* and *Streptococcus* spp. in the fecal samples from the CFS group (3.5 x 10(7) cfu [colony forming units]/L and 9.8 x 10(7) cfu/L respectively) were significantly higher than those for the control group (5.0 x 10(6) cfu/L and 8.9 x 10(4) cfu/L respectively). [**Note: This is approximately a 7x increase in D-lactate producing *Enterococcus* and 1,100x increase in D-lactate producing *Streptococcus*.**] Analysis of exometabolic profiles of *Enterococcus faecalis* and *Streptococcus sanguinis*, representatives of *Enterococcus* and *Streptococcus* spp. respectively, by NMR and HPLC showed that these organisms produced significantly more lactic acid from (13)C-labeled glucose, than the Gram negative *Escherichia coli*. Further, **both *E. faecalis* and *S. sanguinis* secrete more D-lactic acid than *E. coli*.** This study suggests a probable link between intestinal colonization of Gram-positive facultative anaerobic D-lactic acid bacteria and symptom expressions in a subgroup of patients with CFS. Given the fact that **this might explain not only neurocognitive dysfunction in CFS patients but also mitochondrial dysfunction, these findings may have important clinical implications**."

Patients with "chronic fatigue syndrome" and the associated neurologic dysfunction and muscle dysfunction have intestinal overgrowth of bacteria that produce D-lactic acid, a known neurotoxin and metabolic poison

In 2007 and 2008, the current author (AV) wrote and published *Musculoskeletal Pain: Expanded Clinical Strategies** with the Institute for Functional Medicine; this chapter on fibromyalgia is derived and updated from that work. In that publication, I reviewed evidence that fibromyalgia—at that time considered mysterious, idiopathic, chronic, relentless, and treatable only by pain-relieving drugs—was most likely caused by small intestine bacterial overgrowth (SIBO) and the resultant absorption of metabolic toxins and immunogenic debris. This perspective has been supported by numerous publications, particularly the article published by Sheedy et al** in 2009, which showed for the first time that patients with chronic fatigue syndrome—a condition tightly correlated with and which often overlaps with fibromyalgia—have SIBO with various bacteria that are high-output producers of D-lactic acid, a known neurotoxin and metabolic poison which potentially contributes to many of the main clinical, biochemical, and histologic manifestations of FM, namely mental fatigue and dyscognition (difficulty thinking), muscle fatigue and pain, biochemical evidence of mitochondrial impairment, and histologic evidence of mitochondrial myopathy.

*Vasquez A. *Musculoskeletal Pain: Expanded Clinical Strategies*. Institute for Functional Medicine, 2008.
**Sheedy JR, Wettenhall RE, Scanlon D, et al. Increased d-lactic acid intestinal bacteria in patients with chronic fatigue syndrome. *In Vivo*. 2009 Jul-Aug;23(4):621-8

---

4. Bacterial LPS and other antigens absorbed from the intestine during SIBO contribute to a subclinical inflammatory state that results in pain hypersensitivity and increased cytokine release, both of which are characteristics of fibromyalgia: In animal models and in human research studies, exposure to bacterial endotoxin/LPS has been shown to increase the brain's sensitivity to and perception of pain. Immune-mediated and inflammation-mediated pathways that promote pain sensitivity and pain perception include ❶ reduced production of nitric oxide with ❷ increased production of prostaglandins and cytokines, resulting in ❸ the sensitization of peripheral and/or central neurons to pain perception/transmission. In support of this concept, Lin[123] wrote in 2004, "**The immune response to bacterial antigen in SIBO provides a framework for understanding the hypersensitivity in both fibromyalgia and IBS.**" A later paper by Othmanm, Agüero, and Lin[124] in 2008 stated, "…a recent animal study demonstrated that exposure to endotoxin increased the production of

prostaglandins and simultaneously decreased nitrous oxide production, resulting in inflammatory hyperalgesia" and "These observations suggest that SIBO is a common feature in both [IBS and FM] disorders and that altered gut microbiota in SIBO may play a role in the induction of somatic or visceral hypersensitivity, with affected patients meeting the diagnostic criteria for IBS, fibromyalgia or both disorders."

5. <u>Central sensitization (enhanced and autonomous pain hypersensitivity) seen in FM can be caused by bacterial LPS</u>: Somewhat independent from the immune/inflammation-mediated hyperalgesia induced by LPS is the hyperalgesia mediated by central nervous system responses. The central sensitization seen with fibromyalgia[125] might be explained as being caused by intestinally-derived bacterial toxins. **Bacterial LPS/endotoxin promotes central sensitization via direct activation of NMDA receptors and by inducing hyperalgesia (elevated pain perception)**

Exposure to the bacterial endotoxin lipopolysaccharide (LPS) causes increased sensitivity to painful stimuli (hyperalgesia) and a reduction in opioid analgesia (anti-analgesia)
"Intraperitoneal injection of toxins, such as the bacterial endotoxin lipopolysaccharide (LPS), is associated with a well-characterized increase in sensitivity to painful stimuli (hyperalgesia) and a longer-lasting reduction in opioid analgesia (anti-analgesia) when pain sensitivity returns to basal levels."
Johnston IN, Westbrook RF. Inhibition of morphine analgesia by LPS: role of opioid and NMDA receptors and spinal glia. *Behav Brain Res.* 2005 Jan

and anti-analgesia (reduced response to pain inhibition).[126] Accumulated evidence suggests that fibromyalgia may be a disorder of somatic hypersensitivity induced by bacterial toxins derived from quantitative excess or qualitative abnormalities in gut bacteria.[127]

6. <u>SIBO commonly causes nutrient malabsorption and thus leads to malnutrition</u>: SIBO causes nutrient malabsorption[128] and can thereby contribute to the vitamin D and magnesium deficiencies that promote pain and mitochondrial dysfunction, respectively, and which are common in fibromyalgia. Intestinal bacterial overgrowth causes nutrient malabsorption via intestinal inflammation and villus atrophy (anatomic impairment) and impairment of digestion, specifically the enzymatic degradation of mucosal peptidases and disaccharidases by bacterial proteases (biochemical impairment). As reported by McEvoy and

colleagues[129], bacterial contamination [overgrowth] of the small intestine is an important cause of occult malabsorption and malnutrition, especially in the elderly.

7. <u>SIBO can be triggered or exacerbated by emotional stress</u>: SIBO can be triggered in humans by reduced mucosal immunity following stressful life events, and this helps explain the link between psychoemotional stress and the SIBO-related conditions IBS and FM. Chronic mental-emotional stress causes reduced production of the antibody secretory IgA (sIgA) which is the primary line of defense against bacteria and other microorganisms in the gastrointestinal tract; thus, mental-emotional stress can reduce intestinal immunity and thereby promote bacterial overgrowth in the intestines.

8. <u>Oxidative stress triggers exaggerated pain perception— hyperalgesia (hypersensitivity to pain) and allodynia (perception of pain from normal stimuli)</u>: Patients with fibromyalgia show evidence of increased free radical (oxidant) production and reduced antioxidant defenses. Increased oxidative stress can be caused by immune activation and mitochondrial dysfunction; immune activation and mitochondrial dysfunction also promote oxidative stress and depletion of antioxidants, resulting in a vicious cycle, as illustrated in the diagram below.

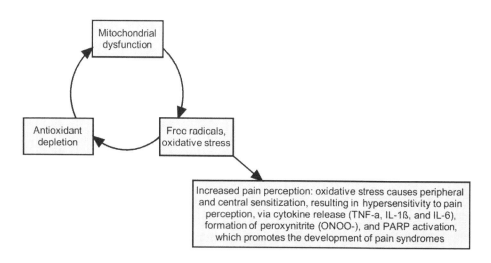

Mitochondrial dysfunction increases free radical production, which promotes hypersensitivity to pain perception

In the excellent review by Cordero et al[130], the authors note that recent studies have shown that oxidative stress causes peripheral and central sensitization and alters nerve sensitivity to pain (nociception), resulting in hyperalgesia—hypersensitivity to normal stimuli. The free radical (oxidant) superoxide promotes the development of pain through direct peripheral sensitization and the release of various cytokines (such as TNF-α, IL-1β, and IL-6), the formation of peroxynitrite (ONOO-), and PARP activation. PARP—poly-ADP-ribose-polymerase—is a nuclear enzyme activated by superoxide/peroxynitrite radicals; activation of PARP promotes the development of pain syndromes, including the components of small sensory fiber neuropathy, thermal and mechanical hyperalgesia, tactile allodynia, and exaggerated pain behavior in animal models of diabetic neuropathy.[131,132]

9. <u>Low plasma levels of L-tryptophan seen in fibromyalgia patients can be caused by degradation of dietary tryptophan by the bacterial enzyme tryptophanase</u>: Patients with fibromyalgia have low blood levels of the amino acid L-tryptophan[133], which is used in the body to make serotonin (important for mood maintenance and pain alleviation) and melatonin (important for normal sleep and for support of mitochondrial function and antioxidant protection). Bacteria such as *Escherichia coli, Proteus vulgaris,* and *Bacteroides* produce the enzyme tryptophanase[134], which destroys L-tryptophan in the gut before it is absorbed from ingested foods; thus, generalized bacterial overgrowth of the small intestine could reasonably be expected to exacerbate this phenomenon. In patients with fibromyalgia, higher tryptophan levels correlate positively with serotonin levels and with less pain and better sleep, while lower tryptophan levels are associated with sleep impairment, reduced serotonin levels, and higher levels of substance P, a neurotransmitter that promotes inflammation and pain perception.[135] Fibromyalgia patients produce 31% less melatonin than do healthy controls, and "this may contribute to impaired sleep at night, fatigue during the day, and changed pain perception."[136] Thus, a likely sequence of events is that, for example, a period of stressful life events can cause impair gastrointestinal immunity leading to intestinal bacterial overgrowth, which itself causes tryptophan degradation via elaboration of bacterial tryptophanase, causing tryptophan deficiency and resultant deficiencies of serotonin (leading to pain, depression, anxiety, and food/carbohydrate craving) and melatonin

(leading to sleep disturbance, impaired antioxidant defense and mitochondrial function, and impaired immune responsiveness).

10. The therapies that help fibromyalgia share mechanisms of action consistent with the model presented here: As will be reviewed below under *Therapeutic Interventions*, essentially all of the most successful therapies for fibromyalgia have effects on intestinal flora, muscle perfusion/contractility, or mitochondrial bioenergetics (biological production of cellular energy/ATP). This is true for vegetarian diets (which favorably alter gut flora and improve antioxidant defenses), supplementation with tryptophan/melatonin (which preserve mitochondrial function during bacterial LPS/endotoxin exposure), physical treatments such as acupuncture (which improves tissue perfusion), and the use of nutrients such as magnesium, acetyl-L-carnitine, D-ribose, creatine, and coenzyme Q-10—all of which support or improve mitochondrial function.

11. Restless leg syndrome and fibromyalgia commonly co-exist, and restless leg syndrome can be alleviated by eradication of SIBO: Restless leg syndrome (RLS) occurs in approximately 30% of FM patients and can be effectively treated by addressing SIBO with a combination of antibiotics (drugs or botanical medicines that eradicate bacteria) and probiotics (products containing beneficial bacteria, which help restore "microbial balance" in the gastrointestinal tract).[137]

12. Antimicrobial/antibiotic treatment alleviates fibromyalgia in most FM patients, just as it also alleviates gastrointestinal symptoms in patients with irritable bowel syndrome (IBS): Finally and most importantly, **antimicrobial therapy alleviates FM (and IBS) symptoms in direct proportion to the success of bacterial overgrowth eradication**, thus adding strong direct evidence in support of SIBO as a main cause of FM.[138,139] Recent clinical trials have shown that treatment of the fibromyalgia-related conditions IBS and SIBO by use of the nonabsorbed oral antibiotic rifaximin results in significant diminution of IBS-SIBO symptomatology with benefits lasting after the discontinuation of therapy.[140,141]

  ▫ Clinical trial: Rifaximin therapy for patients with irritable bowel syndrome without constipation (*New England Journal of Medicine* 2011 Jan[142]): Authors of this study evaluated rifaximin, a minimally absorbed antibiotic, as treatment for IBS. Subjects were given rifaximin at a dose of 550 mg or placebo, three times daily for 2 weeks and were followed for

10 weeks thereafter. "Significantly more patients in the rifaximin group than in the placebo group had adequate relief of global IBS symptoms during the first 4 weeks after treatment (40.8% vs. 31.2%). Similarly, more patients in the rifaximin group than in the placebo group had adequate relief of bloating (39.5% vs. 28.7%). In addition, significantly more patients in the rifaximin group had a response to treatment as assessed by daily ratings of IBS symptoms, bloating, abdominal pain, and stool consistency. The incidence of adverse events was similar in the two groups." Thus, among patients who had IBS without constipation, treatment with rifaximin for 2 weeks provided significant relief of IBS symptoms, bloating, abdominal pain, and loose or watery stools. *Comments by Dr Vasquez: Shortcomings of the intervention used in this IBS-rifaximin study include ❶ failure to use long-term treatment, which is often necessary in the treatment of chronic SIBO, ❷ failure to co-administer an antifungal agent to avert fungal growth in the intestines which commonly occurs as a result of antimicrobial/antibacterial drug treatment, ❸ failure to administer probiotics to re-establish beneficial flora, and ❹ failure to implement dietary modification to sustain the beneficial eradication of excess bacteria—allowing patients to continue their unhealthy diets and lifestyles is the most assured way to ensure that the condition (SIBO-IBS) will return.*

▫ Review of clinical trials: Rifaximin as treatment for SIBO and IBS (*Expert Opinion on Investigational Drugs* 2009 Mar[143]): A recognized expert in the treatment of SIBO-related conditions, Dr Pimentel writes, "**Rifaximin is a broad-range, gastrointestinal-specific antibiotic that demonstrates no clinically relevant bacterial resistance**. Therefore, rifaximin may be useful in the treatment of gastrointestinal disorders associated with altered bacterial flora, including irritable bowel syndrome (IBS) and small intestinal bacterial overgrowth (SIBO)." He also notes regarding the use of rifaximin in the treatment of IBS, "Rifaximin improved global symptoms in 33 - 92% of patients and eradicated SIBO in up to 84% of patients with IBS, with results sustained up to 10 weeks post-treatment. Rifaximin caused a lower number of adverse events compared with metronidazole or levofloxacin and may have a more favorable adverse event profile than systemic antibiotics, without clinically relevant antibiotic resistance."

- Results of two clinical trials of antibiotics in the treatment of fibromyalgia: Fibromyalgia—the gastrointestinal link (*Current Pain and Headache Reports* 2004 Oct[144]): This article discusses the results of two experiments using antibiotics in the treatment of FM: ❶ 96 patients with SIBO diagnosed by lactulose hydrogen breath testing (LHBT) were offered antibiotic treatment for the reduction of gastrointestinal bacteria; 25 of the 96 patients returned for a follow-up LHBT. Neomycin was the most commonly used antibiotic. Eleven of the 25 patients achieved complete transient eradication of SIBO after antibiotic treatment and experienced better improvement in more of their FM symptom scores when compared with the patients who did not achieve complete eradication. This indicates that **a direct relationship exists between the presence of SIBO and intestinal and extraintestinal symptoms in fibromyalgia, and that FM can be alleviated by effective antimicrobial/antibiotic treatment**. ❷ In this double-blind trial of eradication of SIBO in fibromyalgia, 46 patients fulfilling the established criteria for FM were tested for SIBO using LHBT. Forty-two of the 46 patients (91.3%) were positive for SIBO and were randomized to receive placebo or 500 mg of liquid neomycin (a minimally-absorbed gastrointestinal-specific antibiotic drug) twice daily for 10 days. Only six of the 20 patients (30%) in the neomycin group achieved eradication (indicating inefficacy of treatment); thus, no statistically significant difference between groups was available for analysis. Thereafter, 28 patients in the double-blind study testing positive for SIBO went on to receive open-label antibiotic treatment to eradicate SIBO, and this time 17 of the 28 patients (60.7%) achieved eradication of SIBO. When these 23 patients were compared with the 15 patients who failed to eradicate or did not undergo open-label treatment, significant improvement attributable to antibiotic treatment in the FM scores was detected. **Results suggest that eradication of bacterial overgrowth results in a statistically and clinically significant alleviation of FM symptoms.**

Thus, overall and when integrated together, the research literature provides compelling evidence linking intestinal bacterial overgrowth with the genesis and perpetuation of fibromyalgia. Chronic low-dose exposure to bacterial debris such as lipopolysaccharide/endotoxin and metabolic toxins such as hydrogen sulfide and D-lactic acid from SIBO is a plausible cause of impaired cellular energy production that results in chronic, widespread muscle fatigue and soreness and which may culminate in the clinical presentation of fibromyalgia. The individual components of this model have been substantiated by mechanistic studies in animals and/or research studies in humans. CFS also shares many epidemiological and clinical similarities with FM, and a similar pathophysiology is highly probable.

A consistent report from many CFS and fibromyalgia patients is that of environmental intolerance (EI) and multiple chemical sensitivity (MCS), often grouped together as EI-MCS; these are complex disorders that the medical profession has failed to appreciate and which are characterized by adverse physiological responses to ambient levels of toxic chemicals and other environmental exposures. EI-MCS can be plausibly explained by SIBO because bacterial LPS/endotoxin impairs hepatic cytochrome P450 detoxification enzymes, resulting in reduced drug metabolism and impaired clearance of xenobiotics/toxins.[145] Accumulation of xenobiotics in CFS patients[146] might therefore be explained in part by LPS-induced inhibition of xenobiotic clearance secondary to SIBO. Further, the metabolic and immunologic effects of LPS can also account for the immune activation, neurological dysfunction, and musculoskeletal complaints noted in patients with CFS, IBS, and FM. A simplified yet accurate model of fibromyalgia which accounts for the major clinical and objective abnormalities seen with this condition is presented in the diagram that follows. Following the exclusion of diagnosable and treatable conditions that can contribute to or mimic fibromyalgia, and by using an integrated model of functional medicine clinicians can design treatment plans based on the previously reviewed pathogenesis and on the therapeutic considerations detailed in the following section.

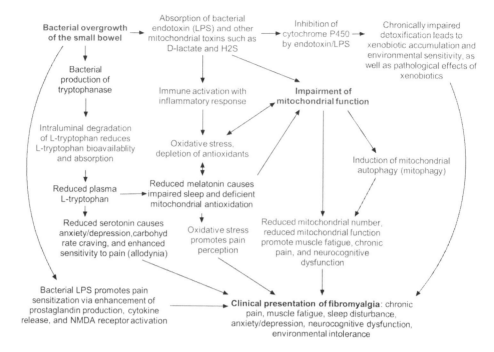

How small intestine bacterial overgrowth (SIBO) causes fibromyalgia: Bacterial overgrowth of the small bowel leads to chronic low-grade tryptophan insufficiency resulting in reduced endogenous production of serotonin (important for positive mood and relief from anxiety pain) and of melatonin (important for restful sleep and protection of mitochondria from oxidative stress). Bacterial "metabolic-mitochondrial toxins" such as endotoxin and D-lactate cause impaired mitochondrial energy production, which leads to mitophagy, muscle fatigue, pain, and cognitive impairment.

Therapeutic Interventions

- **Overview**: Treatments for FM should be ❶ science-based and should ❷ directly address the cause(s) of the disorder; treatments should be ❹ safe (generally) and ❺ effective and ❻ without potential for serious adverse effects. Drug treatment of FM does not meet these criteria; the integrative, nutritional, and functional medicine approaches outlined below can—when properly employed by a skilled clinician—address the cause(s) of FM in a way that is scientific, direct, safe, effective, and well tolerated by essentially all patients. **Treatments for FM must emphasize eradication of SIBO, prevention of SIBO recurrence, the restoration/establishment of optimal nutritional status, and specific support for optimal mitochondrial function; anything less than this will fail to be effective.** Clinical interventions for the treatment of SIBO include dietary carbohydrate restriction, normalization of slow gastrointestinal transit time (e.g., correction of hypothyroidism), selective use of probiotic supplements to normalize intestinal flora, support of mucosal immunity (with nutrients such as vitamin A, zinc, and L-glutamine), and eradication of bacterial overgrowth with drugs (such as ciprofloxacin, rifaximin, amoxicillin/Augmentin[147], metronidazole) and/or natural products (such as berberine[148], *Artemisia annua*, peppermint oil[149], and emulsified time-released oil of oregano[150])—each of these have been reviewed in greater detail elsewhere by this author.[151] Failure of any monotherapeutic approach to immediately resolve the clinical manifestations of FM can explained by the secondary metabolic, immune, and neurophysiological effects that have generally persisted over periods ranging from years to decades for most patients; in other words, the treatment program must be multifaceted in order to address the numerous major problems that cause FM, and the treatment plan must also be sustained long enough to correct the abnormal physiologic patterns that have been established by the body's response/adaptation to the disease process. The treatment program (examples provided) must be complete in order to facilitate correction of systemic oxidative damage (broad-spectrum antioxidant support), resultant nutritional deficiencies (diet optimization, vitamin and mineral supplementation), immune sensitization and induction of proinflammatory cycles (anti-inflammatory nutrition), alterations in neurotransmission and membrane receptor function (amino acid and fatty acid supplementation), and the inflammation-induced disturbances in pain reception and hypothalamic-pituitary-endocrine function (assess/correct hormonal imbalances; supplement with n-3 fatty acids and olive oil to reduce hypothalamic inflammation[152], etc.). Further, patients treated for SIBO who do not positively change their diets and lifestyles (which probably promoted the genesis and perpetuation of the disease-causing SIBO in the first place) are subject to continual recurrence until such changes are implemented and faithfully maintained.

- **Diet optimization with the five-part "supplemented Paleo-Mediterranean Diet"**: The "supplemented Paleo-Mediterranean Diet" (SPMD)—the 5-part nutritional wellness protocol—as described in most of my textbooks in "chapter 2" and also in my articles available on-line at http://optimalhealthresearch.com/protocol.html should be implemented for most FM patients; exceptions to this general rule might include patients with renal insufficiency due to the risk for potassium excess (hyperkalemia[Note 153]). Because any patient might have an allergy or intolerance to any food (even a healthy food like citrus fruit, chicken or eggs), patients and doctors must be aware of the potential for food allergies and will therefore have to customize the Paleo-Mediterranean diet *for each* *individual patient* to exclude foods to which the patient might be allergic or sensitive/intolerant. Otherwise, this 5-part nutrition protocol is based on ❶ fruits, vegetables, nuts, seeds, berries and lean sources of protein, ❷ high-potency multivitamin and multimineral supplementation, ❸ physiologic doses of vitamin D3 to optimize blood levels of vitamin D3 (measured as 25-OH-vitamin D), ❹ combination fatty acid supplementation (with flax oil [for ALA], fish oil [for EPA and DHA], and borage oil [for GLA] with oleic acid from olive oil incorporated into the diet), and ❺ probiotics—foods or supplements that contain living bacteria with beneficial qualities. The diet should emphasize strict avoidance of grains in general and gluten-containing grains *especially wheat* in particular. This diet is essential for the provision of sufficient protein, fiber, phytonutrients, and alkalinization—potassium citrate is most concentrated in vegetables and helps the body maintain proper acid-alkaline balance.[154] The diet should be low in carbohydrates to reduce fermentable substrate to intestinal bacteria. The most important books for patients to read in support of this diet are *The Paleo Diet* by

> **Patients with migraine headaches often have food allergies/sensitivities/intolerances**
>
> "The commonest foods causing reactions were wheat (78%), orange (65%), eggs (45%), tea and coffee (40% each), chocolate and milk (37%) each), beef (35%), and corn, cane sugar, and yeast (33% each). When an average of ten common foods were avoided there was a dramatic fall in the number of headaches per month, 85% of patients becoming headache-free."
>
> Grant EC. Food allergies and migraine. *Lancet.* 1979 May

Dr Loren Cordain and *Breaking the Vicious Cycle* by Elaine Gottschall; an open-access summary of the diet plan is available at OptimalHealthResearch.com/spmd.html.

- o Vegetarian diet: Fibromyalgia syndrome improved using a mostly raw vegetarian diet (*BMC Complementary and Alternative Medicine* 2001 Sep[155]): Diets high in fruits, vegetables, nuts, berries, and seeds provide ample fiber to promote laxation and can be useful as adjunctive treatment for gastrointestinal dysbiosis in general and SIBO in particular (i.e., *quantitative* reduction in GI dysbiosis). Perhaps more importantly, plant-based diets result in *qualitative* benefits by changing microbial behavior and reducing production of irritants, toxins, and bacterial metabolites, including the mitochondrial poisons D-lactate and hydrogen sulfide. Fibromyalgia patients who consume a mostly vegetarian diet have experienced significant improvements in function and reductions in FM symptomatology. Poorly designed dietary interventions that allow abundant intake of whole-grain bread, pasta, rice, and fruit juice[156] would be expected to fail because such high-carbohydrate diets feed intestinal bacteria with an abundance of substrate and would therefore be expected to sustain or exacerbate SIBO. Another advantage to a plant-based mostly-raw diet is the avoidance of dietary advanced glycation end-products (AGEs) which are inflammation-promoting chemical combinations of proteins with sugars, which can be consumed in the diet (e.g., baked deserts) or formed endogenously/internally as a result of oxidative stress and elevated blood sugar levels (e.g., diabetes mellitus). As discussed previously, FM patients show higher levels of AGEs in blood cells and muscle tissue; AGEs promote chronic pain and inflammation[157], and therefore dietary and nutritional strategies that reduce AGE intake and/or AGE formation are 1) without risk, and 2) likely to provide manifold health benefits, including but not limited to reductions in pain and inflammation.

Dr Vasquez's Five-part Nutrition Protocol: The "Supplemented Paleo-Mediterranean Diet"

1. **Diet: Emphasize vegetables, nuts, seeds, berries, and lean sources of protein** (fish, grass-fed lamb/beef). Minimize fruit intake due to higher sugar content while treating SIBO; the goal is to deprive the bacteria and yeast in the intestines of their preferred food source (carbohydrates, sugars). Make modifications for patient-specific food allergies and sensitivities; this is especially important for patients with known allergy-related conditions such as migraine headaches. Patients with kidney disease should use caution when consuming a potassium-rich diet. (Vasquez A. Revisiting the Five-Part Nutritional Wellness Protocol: The Supplemented Paleo-Mediterranean Diet. *Nutritional Perspectives* 2011 Jan)

2. **Multivitamin and multimineral supplement**: Nutrient deficiencies are common and are easily treated with nutritional supplementation. (Fletcher and Fairfield. Vitamins for chronic disease prevention in adults. *JAMA* 2002 Jun)

3. **Vitamin D dosed at 2,000-10,000 IU per day**: The adult requirement for vitamin D3 is approximately 4,000 IU per day; some patients may achieve optimal blood levels with lower doses, but generally daily doses of 4,000-10,000 IU are necessary. (Vasquez A, et al. The Clinical Importance of Vitamin D. *Alternative Therapies in Health and Medicine* 2004 Sep)

4. **Combination fatty acid supplementation**: A combination of flax oil, borage oil, and fish oil provides the health-promoting fatty acids (ALA, GLA, EPA, DHA). Patients should consume organic virgin olive oil liberally with foods. (Vasquez A. New Insights into Fatty Acid Supplementation and Its Effect on Eicosanoid Production and Genetic Expression. *Nutritional Perspectives* 2005; Jan)

5. **Probiotics**: Health-promoting bacteria can be consumed in the form of powders, pills, and fermented foods such as yogurt and kefir.

Note from Dr Vasquez: For additional details and citations to research, please see my other textbooks and the articles I've published and made available on my website http://optimalhealthresearch.com/reprints/series

---

- **Coenzyme Q10 (CoQ-10):** An endogenous antioxidant, vitamin-like substance, and essential component of the mitochondrial electron transport chain, oral supplementation with CoQ-10 has been used therapeutically in numerous studies for the successful treatment of migraine, heart failure, hypertension, and renal failure. Additional data have shown immunomodulatory roles for CoQ-10, and many clinicians employ it as adjunctive treatment for viral infections, cancer, and allergies.[158,159] The electron transport chain is the terminal step in mitochondrial energy/ATP production; as readers can see in the following diagram, each step or "complex" of the electron transport chain requires nutrients, without which energy/ATP production will be impaired, and provision of which (via supplementation) will generally enhance mitochondrial energy/ATP production. **CoQ-10 levels are 40% lower in blood cells of patients with FM compared with levels in healthy persons**, and reduced levels of CoQ-10 correlate with markers associated with expedited destruction of mitochondria (mitophagy).[160]

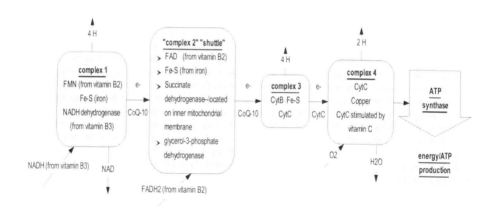

Each step of the mitochondrial electron transport chain requires specific nutrients, without which energy/ATP production cannot proceed: Complex 1 requires vitamin B2 (riboflavin), vitamin B3 (niacin), and CoQ-10. Complex 2 requires vitamin B2 (riboflavin), iron, CoQ-10, and the fatty acid DHA for the function of succinate dehydrogenase. Complex 3 requires iron. Complex 4 requires vitamin C and copper. Step 4 is the enzyme ATP synthase, which produces cellular energy in the form of ATP.

- Clinical investigation: Mitochondrial dysfunction and mitophagy activation in blood mononuclear cells of fibromyalgia patients (*Arthritis Research Therapy* 2010 Jan[161]): The authors studied 2 male and 18 female

FM patients and 10 healthy controls. They evaluated mitochondrial function in blood mononuclear cells from FM patients measuring CoQ-10 levels with high-performance liquid chromatography (HPLC) and measuring mitochondrial membrane potential with flow cytometry. Oxidative stress was determined by measuring mitochondrial superoxide production and lipid peroxidation in blood mononuclear cells and plasma from FM patients. Autophagy activation was evaluated in blood mononuclear cells; mitophagy was confirmed by measuring citrate synthase activity and electron microscopy examination of blood mononuclear cells. The authors **found reduced levels of CoQ-10, decreased mitochondrial membrane potential, increased levels of mitochondrial superoxide in blood mononuclear cells (indicating increased oxidative stress and reduced antioxidant defense),** and increased levels of lipid peroxidation in both blood mononuclear cells and plasma from FM patients. Importantly, the authors note that "mitochondrial dysfunction was also associated with increased expression of autophagic genes and the elimination of dysfunctional mitochondria with mitophagy." *Comment by Dr Vasquez: What this means in practical terms is that the* **biochemical aberrations that cause mitochondrial dysfunction lead to destruction of mitochondria via "mitophagy"** *which literally means "mitochondrial consumption", a process by which dysfunctional mitochondria are eliminated by degradative processes.*

o Clinical trial using a combination of *Ginkgo biloba* and CoQ-10 (*Journal of Internal Medicine Research* 2002 Mar[162]): In an open trial of 23 fibromyalgia patients, the combination of 200 mg CoQ-10 and 200 mg *Ginkgo biloba* (for a total dose of 48 mg flavone glycosides and 12 mg terpene lactones) daily for 84 days was shown to provide clinical benefit in 64% of patients. As noted above, CoQ-10 is often deficient in FM patients, and this deficiency both *causes* and *results from* mitochondrial dysfunction. *Ginkgo biloba* is a botanical/herbal medicine with a long history of human use; the three most important physiologic effects of *Ginkgo biloba* are ❶ vasodilation—improves blood circulation (which is often compromised in FM patients), ❷ improves mitochondrial function and ATP/energy production, and ❸ antioxidant benefits—quenches/absorbs free radicals, which are oxygen-containing molecules that cause damage to cell structures and body tissues. *Comment by Dr Vasquez: Ginkgo biloba and CoQ-10 are very safe and appropriate for use by nearly all FM patients.*

o Case series of FM patients treated with CoQ-10 (*Mitochondrion* 2011 Jul[163]): The authors note that CoQ-10 is an essential electron carrier in the mitochondrial respiratory chain and a strong antioxidant and that **low CoQ-10 levels have been detected in patients with FM**. The authors found that "**FM patients with CoQ-10 deficiency showed a statistically significant reduction in symptoms after CoQ-10 treatment during 9 months (300 mg/day)**. Determination of deficiency and consequent supplementation in FM may result in clinical improvement." *Comment by Dr Vasquez: This is a small but important study documenting 1) that CoQ-10 deficiency is common in FM patients, and 2) that CoQ-10 supplementation alleviates the clinical manifestations/symptoms of FM, consistent with the integrated model of FM presented in this book, which includes the components of nutrient deficiency and mitochondrial dysfunction. Although standardized blood testing for CoQ-10 levels is widely available, testing for and documentation of CoQ-10 deficiency is not necessary before the use of CoQ-10 supplementation.*

o <u>Clinical investigation and clinical trial: Oxidative stress, headache symptoms in fibromyalgia and the role of CoQ-10 in clinical improvement</u> (*PLoS One* 2012 Apr[164]): The authors introduce this study by noting that FM is a chronic pain syndrome with "unknown etiology" and a wide spectrum of symptoms such as allodynia (perception of pain from stimuli that are not normally painful), debilitating fatigue, joint stiffness, and migraine headaches. The authors note a link between oxidative stress and the clinical symptoms in FM. In this study, the researchers examined oxidative stress and bioenergetic status in blood mononuclear cells (BMCs) and the association with headache symptoms in FM patients. Following this correlative analysis, the authors assessed the effects of oral CoQ-10 supplementation on biochemical markers and clinical improvements. In 20 FM patients and 15 healthy controls, a variety of validated clinical and biochemical parameters was assessed; specifically for the biochemical component, measurements were performed for serum CoQ-10, catalase, lipid peroxidation (LPO) levels and ATP levels in BMCs. In patients with FM, the authors found lower CoQ-10 (CoQ-10 deficiency), lower catalase (reduced antioxidant defenses) and lower ATP levels (reduced energy production) in BMCs while FM patients also showed elevated LPO (evidence of free-radical damage) in BMCs. Lower levels of CoQ-10 and catalase levels in BMCs correlated with greater severity-frequency of headache. **In this clinical trial using CoQ-10 300 mg/d for 3 months, CoQ-10 supplementation caused significant reductions in pain and tender points, significant reductions in headache impact, significant elevations in cellular levels of CoQ-10, a reduction in malondialdehyde (marker of lipid** peroxidation) from 30nmol to 5 nmol (normal 6 nmol), an increase in catalase levels from 35 U/mg to 85 U/mg (normal 96 U/mg), and an increase in BMC production of ATP/energy from 61 nmol/mg to 191 nmol/mg (normal 202 nmol/mg). Supplementation with CoQ-10 300 mg/day divided in three doses for 3 months "restored biochemical parameters and induced a significant improvement in clinical and headache symptoms." *Note by Dr Vasquez: The dose of CoQ-10 used clinically is generally approximately 100 mg per day, and occasionally a patient or doctor might decide to use a higher dose, which might be up to 300 mg per day.*

- **Tryptophan and 5-hydroxytryptophan (5-HTP):** Tryptophan is an amino acid found in many foods and is essential for human health and survival. Tryptophan is available as a nutritional supplement only by a doctor's prescription; it is available over-the-counter in a nonprescription supplement in the form of 5-hydroxytryptophan (5-HTP), which is commonly sourced from the seeds of *Griffonia simplicifolia*, a woody climbing shrub native to West and Central Africa. Tryptophan is the precursor to the neurotransmitter serotonin, which has antidepressant, anti-anxiety, and analgesic properties. Patients with FM are known to have low blood levels (i.e., functional nutritional insufficiency) of tryptophan, and the severity of the deficiency correlates with the severity of pain.[165,166,167] Blood levels of serotonin are often below normal in FM patients.[168] The accepted *medical-pharmacological* use of selective serotonin reuptake inhibitors (SSRI) drugs to treat the pain, depression, and anxiety associated with FM supports the use of 5-HTP to raise serotonin levels *naturally* by correcting the underlying nutritional insufficiency. As an over-the-counter nutritional supplement, the 5-hydroxylated form of tryptophan (5-HTP) has been used clinically and in numerous research studies. **Supplementation with 5-HTP has been shown to significantly alleviate symptoms of fibromyalgia.**[169] Commonly used doses range from 50 to 300 mg/d, with larger doses divided throughout the day. If tryptophan rather than 5-HTP is used, results are improved when taken on an empty stomach with carbohydrate (such as honey or fruit juice) to induce insulin secretion, which preferentially promotes uptake of tryptophan into the brain. Deficiency of either magnesium or vitamin B6 impairs conversion of 5-HTP into serotonin, and therefore the interventional program must ensure nutritional supra-sufficiency.
  - o Primary fibromyalgia syndrome and 5-hydroxy-L-tryptophan: a 90-day open study (*Journal of Internal Medicine Research* 1992 Apr[170]): An open 90-day study in 50 fibromyalgia patients showed significant improvement in all measured parameters (number of tender points,

anxiety, pain intensity, quality of sleep, fatigue) after treatment with 5-HTP; global clinical improvement assessed by the patient and the investigator indicated a "good" or "fair" response in nearly 50% of the patients during the treatment period.

- o *Double-blind study of 5-hydroxytryptophan versus placebo in the treatment of primary fibromyalgia syndrome* (*Journal of Internal Medicine Research* 1990 May-Jun[171]): A double-blind, placebo-controlled study using 5-HTP in 50 fibromyalgia patients showed significant improvement in all measured parameters, with only mild and transient side effects. *Note by Dr Vasquez: Again, the common dose range for 5-HTP is 50 to 300 mg per day with doses greater than 100 mg generally best divided throughout the day (e.g., 50 mg thrice per day). I generally recommend starting with 50-100 mg about one hour before bedtime, then adding incremental additions of 50 mg throughout the day for a maximum daily dose of 300 mg. Effectiveness is increased with additional supplementation with magnesium, vitamin B6 (pyridoxine), and the fatty acids found in fish oil (EPA and DHA).*

- **Melatonin:** Melatonin is a hormone produced in the pineal gland of the brain; melatonin is synthesized from the neurotransmitter serotonin, and production of both serotonin and melatonin are dependent on the nutritional availability of tryptophan and/or 5-HTP as discussed above. Patients with FM show decreased nocturnal secretion of melatonin.[172] Melatonin benefits FM patients through a wide range of mechanisms, including promotion of restful sleep and reduction in LPS-induced mitochondrial impairment. As a powerful antioxidant, melatonin scavenges oxygen and nitrogen-based reactants generated in mitochondria and thereby limits the loss of intramitochondrial glutathione, the most important component of antioxidant defense; this prevents damage to mitochondrial protein and DNA. **Melatonin increases the activity of Complexes 1 and 4 of the mitochondrial electron transport chain, improving mitochondrial respiration and increasing ATP synthesis** under various physiological and experimental conditions.[173] Successful treatment with melatonin or its precursor tryptophan/5-HTP should not deter the clinician from addressing other contributing or causative problems such as vitamin D deficiency, gastrointestinal dysbiosis including SIBO, magnesium deficiency, and chronic psychoemotional stress. The adult physiologic dose which mimics natural internal (endogenous) production is approximately 200-500 mcg [micrograms] nightly. In adults, supplementation with melatonin has a wide therapeutic index and has been used safely and effectively in doses up to 20 to 40 mg [milligrams] nightly.

- o Case series (n=4): Melatonin therapy in fibromyalgia (*Journal of Pineal Research* 2006 Jan[174]): Melatonin (3–6 mg per night, administered orally 1 hour before bedtime) has been reported to normalize sleep, alleviate pain and fatigue, and resolve many other clinical manifestations of FM. The authors report, "After 15 days of treatment with melatonin, all patients developed a sleep/wake cycle that was considered normal. They also mentioned a significant reduction of pain. At this time, the patients were taken off hypnotics. Thirty days after the initiation of melatonin, other medications were withdrawn and thereafter they only took melatonin." *Comment by Dr Vasquez: These results are impressive, but—again—the other components of FM such as SIBO and CoQ-10 deficiency should also be treated assertively to reduce the risk of relapse and to treat the underlying problems; good healthcare and good selfcare should extend beyond mere symptom alleviation.*

- o Clinical trial (n=101): Adjuvant use of melatonin for treatment of fibromyalgia (*Journal of Pineal Research*. 2011 Apr[175]): group A (24 patients) treated with 20 mg/day fluoxetine alone; group B (27 patients) treated with melatonin 5 mg alone; group C (27 patients) treated with 20 mg fluoxetine plus 3 mg melatonin; group D (23 patients) treated with 20 mg fluoxetine plus 5 mg melatonin for 8 weeks. "Using melatonin (3 mg or 5 mg/day) in combination with 20 mg/day fluoxetine resulted in significant reduction in both total and different components of Fibromyalgia Impact Questionnaire score compared to the pretreatment values. In conclusion, **administration of melatonin, alone or in a combination with fluoxetine, was effective in the treatment of patients with FMS**."

- **Magnesium:** Magnesium deficiency is epidemic in industrialized societies due to insufficient dietary intake (e.g., from mineral water and leafy green vegetables) and concomitant metabolic-urinary acidosis, which increases urinary magnesium loss.[176,177] Additional causes of magnesium deficiency in fibromyalgia patients include vitamin D deficiency, malabsorption due to SIBO, and the stress of chronic illness. Magnesium deficiency exacerbates the symptoms of fibromyalgia by contributing to impairment of energy/ATP production in skeletal muscle, increased muscle tone and spasms (hypomagnesemic tetany), and anxiety and increased pain sensitivity—hyperalgesia via NMDA receptor overstimulation and neurocortical hyperexcitability. Magnesium deficiency also promotes constipation and intestinal stasis, which exacerbates SIBO. Magnesium supplementation (600 mg or to bowel tolerance to a limit of 1,500 mg in divided doses [bowel tolerance is defined as the dose—commonly of magnesium or vitamin C—that produces slightly loose stools due to the osmotic laxative effect]) should be used routinely in fibromyalgia patients; the primary cautions with magnesium use are renal insufficiency and the use of magnesium-sparing drugs such as the diuretic drug spironolactone. Modest benefits demonstrated in clinical trials with magnesium and malic acid[178] can easily be exceeded with concomitant interventions to address vitamin D deficiency, SIBO, and mitochondrial dysfunction.

- **Acetyl-L-carnitine (ALC):** Acetyl-L-carnitine is a form of the amino acid L-carnitine, most notable for its critical role in supporting mitochondrial energy/ATP production by supporting the metabolism (beta oxidation) of fatty acids in the mitochondria. A large study with 102 patients showed that ALC (administered by oral and parenteral routes, 1500 mg/d) was beneficial in patients with fibromyalgia.[179] Given the role of ALC in supporting and improving mitochondrial function, this supplement probably benefits fibromyalgia patients by compensating for LPS-induced skeletal muscle dysfunction.

- **D-ribose:** D-ribose is a naturally occurring pentose carbohydrate available as a dietary supplement. When administered orally (5 g thrice daily), it safely provides numerous benefits to fibromyalgia patients, according to a recent pilot study with 41 patients.[180] Improvements are seen in energy, sleep, mental clarity, pain intensity, and well-being, as well as global assessment. Among its beneficial mechanisms of action is enhancement of mitochondrial ATP production. Thus, the benefits of D-ribose supplementation may be mediated by restoration or preservation of mitochondrial impairment caused by LPS in fibromyalgia patients.

- **Creatine monohydrate:** Skeletal muscle levels of phosphocreatine and ATP are reduced in patients with fibromyalgia compared with normal controls; thus, oral supplementation with creatine would appear to be an obvious intervention to restore these depressed levels to normal. Although no formal trials have been conducted, Artimal et al[181] reported that a patient with severe refractory fibromyalgia attained sustained alleviation of depression and pain, as well as improvements in sleep and quality of life, following oral administration of creatine monohydrate for 4 weeks (3 grams daily in the first week, then 5 grams daily). Creatine supplementation has been shown to improve ATP production and oxygen utilization in brain and skeletal muscle in humans.[182]

- *Ginkgo biloba* **extract:** This extract is an extensively researched botanical medicine with a long history of safe and effective clinical use for various conditions, especially those associated with reduced blood flow and impaired mitochondrial function. *Ginkgo biloba* provides antioxidant, anti-inflammatory, vasodilatory, and mitochondrial-protective benefits. Given these therapeutic benefits, *Ginkgo* would appear to be a reasonable therapeutic agent to address the secondary pathophysiology in fibromyalgia. As cited elsewhere, a recent clinical trial using a 2-component treatment that included *Ginkgo* showed benefit in FM patients. *Ginkgo biloba* products are generally standardized for the content of flavone glycosides (approximately 24%) and terpene lactones (approximately 6%) with adult doses ranging from 60-240 mg/d and generally 120 mg/d.

- **Physical modalities (chiropractic, acupuncture, osteopathic manipulation, qigong, balneotherapy):** Chiropractic treatment (including spinal manipulation, stretching, soft tissue treatments, and therapeutic ultrasound) has shown benefit in several fibromyalgia case series and clinical trials.[183,184] Acupuncture (including traditional, nontraditional, and electrical stimulation) also has been found beneficial for fibromyalgia patients.[185,186,187] Acupuncture may relieve fibromyalgia pain by improving regional blood flow, in addition to other mechanisms.[188,189] Because specific needle placement does not appear to be important[190], the conclusion that true acupuncture is ineffective because it may not differ markedly from the results obtained by sham acupuncture[191] may not be logical. A similar conundrum is seen in other clinical trials involving physical interventions such as manual osseous manipulation, wherein authentic treatments and sham treatments may both be effective by virtue of common physiological responses.[192] A short-term trial showed that osteopathic manipulative therapy with standard medical care was superior to medical care alone for FM patients.[193] Qigong was found helpful for 10 fibromyalgia patients, and benefits were still apparent at 3 months' follow-up.[194] In a randomized, controlled clinical trial among 24 female fibromyalgia patients, balneotherapy (bath therapy) in daily 20-minute sessions 5 days per week for 3 weeks (total of 15 sessions; water temperature: 96.8°F = 36°C), resulted in statistically significant reductions in measured inflammatory mediators (PGE2, interleukin-1, LTB4) and amelioration of clinical symptoms among treated FM patients.[195] The symptomatic benefits of balneotherapy for FM patients have been corroborated in other trials.[196,197,198]

- **S-adenosylmethionine (SAMe):** Studies using oral or intravenous administration of the nutritional supplement SAMe have reported conflicting results; however, the overall trend seems to indicate that SAMe (800 mg/d orally) is safe and beneficial in the treatment of fibromyalgia.[199] SAMe helps maintain mitochondrial function by preserving glutathione, and its contribution of methyl groups is important for the regulation of gene expression and neurotransmitter synthesis. *Comment by Dr Vasquez: I do not regularly use this supplement, and I would only use it as a last resort if nothing else had worked or if a particular patient had a specific indication for this supplement.*

- _**Chlorella**_: _Chlorella pyrenoidosa_ is a unicellular green alga that grows in fresh water. It is a dense source of nutrients, particularly vitamin D (500 IU vitamin D per 1.35 g _Chlorella_). _Chlorella_ may have value in treating some fibromyalgia patients, but overall the efficacy is low.[200] Thus, _Chlorella_ should not be used as monotherapy for fibromyalgia, although it may be a useful adjunct either as a source of vitamin D, as a means to help modify gut flora, or as an aid in the detoxification of xenobiotics due to its ability to bind ingested and bile-excreted toxins and prevent their absorption and reabsorption in a manner similar to that of cholestyramine, a drug used to bind cholesterol in the gut, promote its excretion, and thereby lower blood cholesterol levels.[201,202,203] This detoxifying effect of _Chlorella_ in humans is supported by 2 clinical trials showing that nursing mothers who supplement with _Chlorella_ during lactation transfer less dioxin in their breast milk compared to nursing mothers who do not consume _Chlorella_.[204,205]

- **Probiotics:** Probiotics are beneficial bacteria that can be consumed in foods or as nutritional supplements to populate the gut, particularly following antibiotic use or long-term dietary neglect. In addition to their availability in capsules and powders, probiotics are widely consumed in the form of yogurt, kefir, and other cultured foods, and they have an excellent record of safety. Probiotic supplements are available in different strengths (quantity), potencies (viability), and combinations of bacteria (diversity). Some probiotics also contain fermentable carbohydrates (prebiotics) such as fructooligosaccharides (FOS) and inulin, which are substrates to nourish the beneficial bacteria. From a practical clinical perspective, the clinician can choose probiotic foods and supplements and instruct the patient to use these on an ongoing, periodic, or rotational basis. Probiotics (i.e., bacteria only) may have a therapeutic advantage over prebiotics or synbiotics (probiotics+prebiotics) when treating SIBO because the fermentable carbohydrate in prebiotics and synbiotics may exacerbate the preexisting bacterial overgrowth by providing already overpopulated bacteria with additional substrate. The benefits of probiotic supplementation have been demonstrated in patients with IBS,[206,207] rotavirus infection[208], eczema and increased intestinal permeability,[209] and SIBO associated with renal failure.[210] To date, no studies using probiotics in the treatment of fibromyalgia have been published.

Conclusions and Therapeutic Approach

- In sum, current research indicates that fibromyalgia results from impairment of cellular energy/ATP production (mitochondrial dysfunction) and induction of pain hypersensitivity (peripheral and central sensitization) due to absorbed metabolic toxins from bacterial/microbial overgrowth of the gastrointestinal tract; this is complicated by induction of tryptophan deficiency which is most likely caused by tryptophan degradation by bacterial tryptophanase activity and which leads to serotonin and melatonin insufficiencies, which lead to associated biochemical and clinical consequences, discussed previously. Available studies have shown that SIBO is ubiquitous among fibromyalgia patients and that antimicrobial interventions—whether pharmaceutical or nutritional—are efficacious. Secondary physiological effects such as mitochondrial impairment, pain sensitization, nutritional deficiencies, oxidative stress, and reduced tissue perfusion are treated with combined use of select therapeutics as reviewed previously. Patients presenting with widespread pain should be screened for causative underlying disease; if no other explanation can be found, then the diagnosis of fibromyalgia should be made, and the condition should be treated with the nondrug therapeutics discussed above. The first visit can include history, physical examination, and laboratory tests; initial laboratory assessment should include complete blood count (CBC), metabolic/chemistry panel, serum 25-hydroxyvitamin D, C-reactive protein (CRP), anti-nuclear antibodies (ANA), antibodies against cyclic citrullinated proteins (anti-CCP antibodies), ferritin, muscle enzymes aldolase and creatine kinase, and a complete thyroid assessment including TSH, free T4, free T3, total T3, reverse T3 (rT3), and antithyroid peroxidase and antithyroglobulin antibodies. First-day interventions can include dietary optimization, multivitamin-multimineral supplementation (including vitamin D3 and magnesium), tryptophan/5-HTP, CoQ10, mixed tocopherols, and combination fatty acids including gamma-linolenic acid (GLA), eicosapentaenoic acid (EPA) and docosahexaenoic acid (DHA). SIBO can be treated empirically, or it can be objectively assessed with breath hydrogen and methane testing, stool analysis, culture, microscopy, and parasitology. At follow-up visits, additional assessments and interventions (such as for toxic metals and chronic occult infections) can be used to fine-tune the diagnosis and further discover and define its contributors in order to maximize the patient's response to treatment and promote optimal recovery and health.

Format and Layout of this book: The format and layout of this book is designed to efficiently take the reader though the clinically relevant spectrum of considerations for each condition that is detailed. Important topics are given their own section within each chapter, while other less important or less common conditions are only described briefly in terms of the four "clinical essentials" of 1) definition/pathophysiology, 2) clinical presentation, 3) assessment/diagnosis, and 4) treatment/management. Each expanded section which details the more important/common conditions maintains a consistent format, taking the reader through the spectrum of primary clinical considerations: definition/pathophysiology, clinical presentations, differential diagnoses, assessments (physical examination, laboratory, imaging), complications, management, and treatment. As my books have progressed, I am increasingly using an article-by-article review format (especially in the sections on management and treatment) so that readers have more direct access to the information so as to understand and *incorporate* more deeply what the research actually states; the goal and general approach here is to use a *representative sampling* of the research literature.

References and Citations: Citations to articles, abstracts, texts, and personal communications are footnoted throughout the text to provide supporting information and to provide interested readers the resources to find additional information. Many of the cited articles are available on-line for free, and when possible I have included the website addresses so that readers can access the complete article.

Peer-review and Quality Control: Peer-review is essential to help ensure accuracy and clinical applicability of health-related information. Consistent with the importance of our goals, I have employed several "checks and balances" to increase the accuracy and applicability of the information within my textbooks:

- Reliance upon authoritative references: Nearly all important statements are referenced to peer-reviewed biomedical journals or authoritative texts, such as *The Merck Manual* and *Current Medical Diagnosis and Treatment*. Each citation is provided by a footnote at the bottom of each page so that readers will know quickly and easily exactly from where the information was obtained.
- Extensive cross-referencing: Readers will notice, if not be overwhelmed by, the number of references and citations. Many important statements have several references. Many references (especially textbooks) are referenced several times even on the same page. The purpose of this extensive referencing is three-fold: 1) to guide you to additional information, 2) to help me (as writer) stay organized, and 3) to help you and me (the practicing physicians) employ this information with confidence.
- Periodic revision: All of my books will be updated and revised on an *as-needed* basis. New information is added; superfluous information removed. Inspired by the popular text *Current Medical Diagnosis and Treatment* which is updated every year, I want my books to be accurate, timely, and in pace with the ever-growing literature on natural medicine. Any significant errors that are discovered will be posted at OptimalHealthResearch.com/updates; please check this page periodically to ensure that you are working with the most accurate information of which I am aware.

- Peer-review: The peer-review process for my books takes several forms. First, colleagues and students are invited to review new and revised sections of the text before publication; every section of the book that you are holding has been independently reviewed by health science students and/or practicing clinicians from various backgrounds: allopathic, chiropractic, osteopathic, naturopathic. Second, you - the reader - are invited to provide feedback about the information in the book, typographical errors, syntax, case reports, new research, etc. If your ideas truly change the nature of the material, I will be glad to acknowledge you in the text (with your permission, of course). If your contribution is hugely significant, such as reviewing three or more chapters or helping in some important way, I will be glad to not only acknowledge you, but to also send you the next edition at a discount or courtesy when your ideas take effect. Third, I keep abreast of new literature by constantly perusing new research and advancements in the health sciences. Having been successful in three separate doctoral programs in the health sciences, I have learned not only to master large amounts of material but to also separate and integrate different viewpoints as appropriate. I also "field test" my protocols with patients in the various clinical arenas in which I work and also with professionals and academicians via presentations and critical dialogue. By implementing these quality control steps, I hope to create a useful text and advance our professions and our practices by improving the quality of care that we deliver to our patients.

How to Use This Book Safely and Most Effectively: Ideally, these books should be read cover-to-cover within a context of coursework that is supervised by an experienced professor. For post-graduate professionals, they might consider forming a local "book club" and meeting for weekly or monthly discussions to check their understandings and share their clinical experiences to refine the application of clinical knowledge, perceptions, and skills. Virtual groups and internet forums—specifically the forum hosted by the Institute for Functional Medicine at www.FunctionalMedicine.org—can provide access to an assembly of international professional peers wherein sharing of clinical questions and experiences are synergistic. Throughout this book, references are amply provided and are often footnoted with hyperlinks providing full-text access. This book is intended for licensed doctorate-level healthcare professionals with graduate and post-graduate training.

Notice: The intention and scope of this text are to provide doctorate-level clinicians with useful information and a familiarity with available research and resources pertinent to the management of patients in an integrative primary care setting. Specifically, the information in this book is intended to be used by licensed healthcare professionals who have received hands-on clinical training and supervision at accredited health science colleges. Additionally, information in this book should be used in conjunction with other resources, texts, and in combination with the clinician's best judgment and intention to "*first, do no harm*" and second to provide effective healthcare. Information and treatments applicable to a specific *condition* may not be appropriate for or applicable to a specific *patient* in your office; this is especially true for patients with multiple comorbidities and those taking pharmaceutical medications with multiple adverse effects and drug/nutrient/herb interactions. In my books and articles, I describe treatments—manual, dietary, nutritional, botanical, pharmacologic, and occasionally surgical—and their research support for the clinical condition being discussed; each practitioner must determine appropriateness of these treatments for his/her individual patient and with consideration of the doctor's scope of practice, education, training, skill, and—occasionally—the appropriateness of "off label" use of medications and treatments. This book has been carefully written and checked for accuracy by the author and professional colleagues. However, in view of the possibility of human error and new discoveries in the biomedical sciences, neither the author nor any party associated in any way with this text warrants that this text is perfect, accurate, or complete in every way, and we disclaim responsibility for harm or loss associated with the application of the material herein. With all conditions/treatments described herein, each physician must be sure to consider the balance between what is best for the patient and the physician's own level of ability, expertise, and experience. When in doubt, or if the physician is not a specialist in the treatment of a given severe condition, referral is appropriate. These notes are written with the routine "outpatient" in mind and are not tailored to severely injured patients or "playing field" or "emergency response" situations; consult your First Aid and Emergency Response texts and course materials for appropriate information. These notes represent the author's perspective based on academic education, experience, and post-graduate continuing education and are not inclusive of every fact that a clinician may need to know. This is not an "entry level" book except when used in an academic setting with a knowledgeable professor who can explain the concepts, tests, physical exam procedures, and treatments; this book requires a certain level of knowledge from the reader and familiarity with clinical concepts, laboratory assessments, and physical examination procedures.

Updates, Corrections, and Newsletter: When and if omissions, errata, and the need for important updates become clear, I will post these at the website: OptimalHealthResearch.com/updates.html. A reader might access this page periodically to ensure staying informed of any corrections that might have clinical relevance. This book consists not only of the text in the printed pages you are holding, but also the footnotes and any updates at the website. Be alerted to new integrative clinical research and updates to this textbook by signing-up for the free newsletter at www.OptimalHealthResearch.com/newsletter.html.

Language, Semantics, and Perspective: As a diligent student who previously aspired to be an English professor, I have written this text with great (though inevitably imperfect) attention to detail. Individual words were chosen with care. I confess to knowing, pushing, and creatively breaking several rules of grammar and punctuation. With regard to the he/she and him/her debacle of the English language, I've mixed singular and plural pronouns for the sake of being efficient and so that the images remain gender-neutral to the extent reasonable. The subtitle *The art of creating wellness while effectively managing acute and chronic musculoskeletal/health disorders* was chosen to emphasize the intentional creation of wellness rather than a limited focus on disease treatment and symptom suppression. For the 2009 printing of *Chiropractic and Naturopathic Mastery of Common Clinical Disorders*, this subtitle was slightly modified from "creating" to "co-creating" to emphasize the **team effort** required between physician and patient. *Managing* was chosen to emphasize the importance of treating-monitoring-referring-reassessing, rather than merely *treating*. *Disorders* was chosen to reflect the fact that a distinguishing characteristic of *life* is the ability to habitually create *organized structure* and *higher order* from chaos and *disorder*. For example, plants organize the randomly moving molecules of air and water into the organized structure of biomolecules which eventually take shape as plant structure—fiber, leaves, flowers, petals. Similarly, the human body creates organized structure of increased complexity from consumed plants and other foods; molecules ingested and inhaled from the environment are organized into specific biochemicals and tissue structures with distinct characteristics and definite functions. Injury and disease *result in* or *result from* a lack of order, hence my use of the word "disorders" to characterize human illness and disease. A motor vehicle accident that results in bodily injury, for example, is an example of an external chaotic force, which, when imparted upon human body tissues, results in a disruption (disorder) of the normal structure and organization that previously defined and characterized the now-damaged tissues of the body. Likewise, an autoimmune disease process that results in tissue destruction is an *anti-evolutionary* process that takes molecules of higher complexity and reverts them to simpler, fragmented, and non-functional forms. From the perspective of "health" as *organized structure and meaningful function* and "disease" as *the reversion to chaos, destruction of structure, and the loss of function*, the task of healthcare providers is essentially to restore order, and to acutely reduce and proactively prevent/eliminate clinical-biochemical-biomechanical-emotional chaos insofar as it adversely affects the patient's life experience as an individual and our collective experience as an interdependent society. What is required of clinicians then is the ability first to create conceptual order from what appears to be chaotic phenomena, and then second to materialize that conceptual order into our physical world; this is our task, and no small task it is.

Integrity and Creativity: I have endeavored to accurately represent the facts as they have been presented in texts and research, and to specifically resist any temptation to embellish or misrepresent data as others have done.[211,212] Conversely, I have not endeavored to make this book appeal to the "average" student or reader; my goal is to write and teach to the students at the top of the class, thereby affirming them and pulling the other students forward and upward. While I offer *explanations*, I intentionally resist *simplifications*, except when one simplification might facilitate the comprehension of a more complex phenomenon, or when such a simplification might facilitation the conveyance of information from clinician to patient. I have allowed this text to be unique in format, content, and style, so that the personality of this text can be contrasted with that of the instructor and reader, thus enabling the learner to at least benefit from an intentionally different – and intentionally honest – perspective and approach. Students using this text with the guidance of a qualified professor will benefit from the experience of "two teachers" rather than just one.

Linearity, Nonlinearity, Redundancy, Asynchronicity: Although the overall flow of the text is highly linear and sequential, occasionally I place a conclusion before its introduction for the sake of foreshadowing and therefore for preparing the reader for what is to come. The purpose of this is not simply one of preparation for the sake of allowing the reader to know what is already lying ahead on the path, but more to begin creating new "shelf space" in the reader's intellectual-neuronal "library" so that when the new—particularly if *neoparadigmatic*—information is encountered, a space will already exist for it; it other words: the intent is to make learning easier. Likewise, for the sake of *information retention*—or what is better understood as synaptogenesis—important points are presented more than once, either identically or variantly. Given that *"No one ever reads the same book twice"*[213] (because the "person who starts" the reading of a meaningful book is changed into the "person who finishes" the reading of that book (assuming proper intentionality and application of one's "self"), the person reading these words might consider a second glace after the first.

Distinguishing "Integrative Medicine" from "Functional Medicine"—the author's perspective[214]: The distinction of integrative medicine from functional medicine is that of *quantity* from *quality*. Integrative medicine can be understood as a quantitative extension of other already-existing healthcare models, to which additional perspectives and treatments are added; in this way, various conceptual models are "integrated" and used together in a more holistic and comprehensive approach. In contrast, functional medicine is a distinct model of health and disease that has developed an identity beyond mere integration of various models and treatments. Functional medicine is qualitatively distinct in its viewpoint of disease causation and treatment by the unique combination of emphases placed on ❶ patient-centered care (in contrast to the disease-centered care of allopathic medicine and most osteopathic medicine), ❷ detailed appreciation of the importance of the web-like interconnected nature of various organ systems[215] and psychological, physiological, and pathological processes (to a greater extent than allopathic, osteopathic, chiropractic and naturopathic medicine), ❸ its rigorous evidence-based standards, and ❹ its willingness to eagerly-yet-appropriately include *all* therapeutic options, ranging from (for example) surgical to meditative, dietary to pharmaceutical, manipulative to botanical, and antidysbiotic to psychological. In short, functional medicine can be described as an ***antiparadigmatic patient-centered discipline***, hence its therapeutic flexibility, broad applicability, and enhanced efficacy; it is antiparadigmatic due to its lack of adherence to a specific and limited set of tools (most professional disciplines are quite limited in their expertise and scope) and due to the emphasis placed on patient-centered healthcare, which first and always foremost seeks to determine the most efficient path for patient empowerment and healing.

Bon Voyage: All artists and scientists—regardless of genre—grapple with the divergent goals of *perfecting* their work and *presenting* their work; the former is impossible, while the latter is the only means by which the effort can create the desired effect in the world, whether that is pleasure, progress, or both. At some point, we must all agree that it is "good enough" and that it contains the essence of what needs to be communicated. While neither this nor any future edition of this book is likely to be "perfect", I am content with the literature reviewed, presented, and the new conclusions and implications which are described—many for the first time ever—in this text. Particularly for *Integrative Rheumatology* and *Chiropractic and Naturopathic Mastery*, each chapter aims to achieve a paradigm shift which distances us further from the simplistic pharmacocentric model and toward one which authentically empowers both practitioners and patients. With time, I will make future editions more complete and perhaps less polemical—but not less passionate. I hope you are able to implement these conclusions and research findings *into your own life* and into the treatment plans for your patients. In short time, I believe that we will see many of these concepts more broadly implemented. Hopefully this work's value and veracity will promote patients' vitality via the vigilant and virtuous clinicians viewing this volume. To the more attentive and thoroughgoing reader, more is revealed.

Authentic learning is life integration
"Ultimately, no one can extract from things—*books included*—more than he already knows. What one has no access to through experience, one has no ear for."
Friedrich Nietzsche [translated by RJ Hollingdale]. *Ecce Homo: How One Becomes What One Is*. New York & London: Penguin Books; 1979, page 70

Thank you, and I wish you and your patients the best of success and health.

Alex Vasquez, D.C., N.D., D.O.
October 2, 2012

Work as love
"You work that you may keep pace with the earth and the soul of the earth. For to be idle is to become a stranger unto the seasons, and to step out of life's procession. ... Work is love made visible."
Kahlil Gibran (1883-1930). *The Prophet*. Publisher Alfred A. Knopf, 1973

Newsletter & Updates
Be alerted to new integrative clinical research and updates to this textbook by signing-up for the free newsletter, sent several times per year as needed. Join at: www.OptimalHealthResearch.com/newsletter.html

Examples of commonly used abbreviations:

- **25-OH-D** = serum 25-hydroxy-vitamin D(3)
- **ACEi** = angiotensin-2 converting enzyme inhibitor
- **Alpha-blocker** = alpha-adrenergic antagonist
- **ARB** = angiotensin-2 receptor blocker/antagonist
- **ARF** = acute renal failure
- **BB** = beta blocker or beta-adrenergic antagonist
- **BMP** = basic metabolic panel, includes serum Na, K, Cl, CO2, BUN, creatinine, and glucose
- **BP** = blood pressure, **HBP** = high blood pressure
- **BUN** = blood urea nitrogen
- **C&S** = culture and sensitivity
- **CAD** = coronary artery disease
- **CBC** = complete blood count
- **CCB** = calcium channel blocker/antagonist
- **CE** = cardiac enzymes, generally including creatine kinase (CK), creatine kinase myocardial band (CKMB), and troponin-1, with the latter being the most specific serologic marker for acute myocardial injury; for the evaluation of acute MI, these are generally tested 2-3 times at 6-hour intervals with ECG performed at least as often.
- **CHF** = congestive heart failure
- **CHO** = carbohydrate
- **CK** = creatine kinase, historically named creatine phosphokinase (CPK)
- **CKD** = chronic kidney disease, generally stratified into five stages based on GFR of roughly <90, 90-60, 60-30, 30-15, and >15, respectively
- **CMP** = comprehensive metabolic panel, also called a chemistry panel, includes the BMP along with

markers of hepatic status albumin, protein, ALT, AST, may also include alkaline phosphatase and rarely GGT; panels vary per laboratory and hospital.

- **CNS** = central nervous system
- **COPD** = chronic obstructive pulmonary disease
- **CRF**, **CRI** = chronic renal failure/insufficiency
- **CRP** = c-reactive protein, **hsCRP** = high-sensitivity c-reactive protein
- **CT** = computed tomography
- **CVD** = cardiovascular disease
- **CXR** = chest X-ray
- **DM** = diabetes mellitus
- **ECG** or **EKG** = electrocardiograph
- **Echo** = echocardiography
- **GFR** = glomerular filtration rate
- **HDL** = high density lipoprotein cholesterol
- **HTN** = hypertension
- **Ig** = immune globulin = antibodies of the G, A, M, E, or D classes.
- **IHD** = ischemic heart disease
- **IV** = intravenous
- **MCV** = mean cell volume
- **MI** = myocardial infarction
- **MRI** = magnetic resonance imaging, **MRI** = magnetic resonance angiography
- **PRN** = from the Latin "pro re nata" meaning "on occasion" or "when necessary"
- **PTH** = parathyroid hormone, **iPTH** = intact parathyroid hormone
- **PVD** = peripheral vascular disease
- **RA** = rheumatoid arthritis
- **RAD** = reactive airway disease, similar to asthma
- **SLE** = systemic lupus erythematosus
- **TRIG(s)** = serum triglycerides
- **UA** = urinalysis
- **US** = ultrasound

Dosing shorthand (mostly Latin abbreviations): q = each; qd = each day; bid = twice daily; tid = thrice daily; qid = four times per day; po = per os = by mouth; prn = as needed.

Index

1990 ACR guidelines, the diagnosis of fibromyalgia, 13
2010 Fibromyalgia diagnostic criteria—summary and chart for clinical use, 15
2010, new ACR guidelines for the diagnosis and assessment of FM, 14
5-hydroxytryptophan, 55
Abbreviations, 69
acetaminophen, 19
Acetyl-L-carnitine, 58
acupuncture, 59
Amitriptyline, 16
carboxy-methyl-lysine, 11
chiropractic, 59
Chlamydophila pneumoniae, 28
Chlorella, 60
Clinical criteria—description and contrast of the 1990 criteria and the 2010 criteria, 12
Coenzyme Q10, 52
Conclusions and Therapeutic Approach, 60
cosmetics, 32
Creatine monohydrate, 58
Cyclobenzaprine, 19
Cymbalta, 17
detoxification, 32
Diet optimization, 49
dimercaptosuccinic acid, 32
D-lactic acid, 37
DMSA, 32
D-ribose, 58
Duloxetine, 17
Fibromyalgia, 7
fibromyalgia disease, 8
Functional Medicine (FxMed) perspectives, 22
Ginkgo biloba extract, 58
Hemochromatosis, 30
hydrogen sulfide, 37
hypothyroidism, 25
Illustration showing the 9 paired locations of fibromyalgia tender points, 13
iron overload, 30
lead, 31
L-tryptophan, 43
Lyrica, 17
Magnesium, 57
Melatonin, 56
mercurial myopathy, 31
mercury, 31
Milnacipran, 18
mitochondrial dysfunction, 9, 10
mitochondrial myopathy, 9
mitophagy, 10, 39, 48, 52
Mycoplasma species, 28
Occult infections, 28
osteopathic manipulation, 59
Patient (mis)education in standard medicine, 19
pentosidine, 11
Pregabalin, 17
Probiotics, 60
qigong, 59
Restless leg syndrome, 44
Rifaximin, 44
S-adenosylmethionine, 59
Savella, 18
SIBO, 35
Small intestine bacterial overgrowth, 35
Small intestine bacterial overgrowth (SIBO):, 35
Standard Medical Treatment for Fibromyalgia, 16
Therapeutic Interventions, 48
Tramadol, 19
Tryptophan, 55
Vitamin D deficiency, 23
xenobiotics, 31

Notes and citations to research

[1] Ames BN, Elson-Schwab I, Silver EA. High-dose vitamin therapy stimulates variant enzymes with decreased coenzyme binding affinity (increased K(m)): relevance to genetic disease and polymorphisms. *Am J Clin Nutr.* 2002 Apr;75(4):616-58 http://www.ajcn.org/cgi/content/full/75/4/616

[2] Williams RJ. Biochemical Individuality: The Basis for the Genetotrophic Concept. Austin and London: University of Texas Press; 1956

[3] Wilk CA. Medicine, Monopolies, and Malice: How the Medical Establishment Tried to Destroy Chiropractic. Garden City Park: Avery, 1996

[4] Getzendanner S. Permanent injunction order against AMA. *JAMA.* 1988 Jan 1;259(1):81-2 http://optimalhealthresearch.com/archives/wilk.html

[5] Carter JP. Racketeering in Medicine: The Suppression of Alternatives. Norfolk: Hampton Roads Pub; 1993

[6] Morley J, Rosner AL, Redwood D. A case study of misrepresentation of the scientific literature: recent reviews of chiropractic. *J Altern Complement Med.* 2001 Feb;7(1):65-78

[7] Terrett AG. Misuse of the literature by medical authors in discussing spinal manipulative therapy injury. *J Manipulative Physiol Ther.* 1995 May;18(4):203-10

[8] Siegel DM, Janeway D, Baum J. Fibromyalgia syndrome in children and adolescents: clinical features at presentation and status at follow-up. *Pediatrics.* 1998;101(3 Pt 1):377-82

[9] Chakrabarty S, Zoorob R. Fibromyalgia. *Am Fam Physician.* 2007 Jul 15;76(2):247-54

[10] Tierney ML. McPhee SJ, Papadakis MA (eds). Current Medical Diagnosis and Treatment 2006, 45th Edition. New York: Lange Medical Books, pages 820-821

[11] Simms RW. Nonarticular soft tissue disorders. In Andreoli TE, Carpenter CCJ, Griggs RC, and Benjamin IJ (eds). Cecil Essentials of Medicine. Seventh Edition. Philadelphia; Saunders Elsevier, 2007: 851-2

[12] Lin HC. Small intestinal bacterial overgrowth: a framework for understanding irritable bowel syndrome. *JAMA.* 2004 Aug 18;292(7):852-8

[13] "Fibromyalgia is one of the most common chronic pain conditions. The disorder affects an estimated 10 million people in the U.S. and an estimated 3-6% of the world population." National Fibromyalgia Association. http://fmaware.org/PageServera6cc.html?pagename=fibromyalgia_affected Accessed Sept 2012.

[14] Brown MM, Jason LA. Functioning in individuals with chronic fatigue syndrome: increased impairment with co-occurring multiple chemical sensitivity and fibromyalgia. *Dyn Med.* 2007 May 31;6:6 http://www.dynamic-med.com/content/6/1/6

[15] Olsen NJ, Park JH. Skeletal muscle abnormalities in patients with fibromyalgia. *Am J Med Sci.* 1998 Jun;315(6):351-8

[16] Sprott H, Salemi S, Gay RE, et al. Increased DNA fragmentation and ultrastructural changes in fibromyalgic muscle fibres. *Ann Rheum Dis.* 2004 Mar;63(3):245-51

[17] Park JH, Niermann KJ, Olsen N. Evidence for metabolic abnormalities in the muscles of patients with fibromyalgia. *Curr Rheumatol Rep.* 2000 Apr;2(2):131-40

[18] Elvin A, Siosteen AK, Nilsson A, Kosek E. Decreased muscle blood flow in fibromyalgia patients during standardised muscle exercise: a contrast media enhanced colour Doppler study. *Eur J Pain.* 2006 Feb;10(2):137-44

[19] Altindag O, Celik H. Total antioxidant capacity and the severity of the pain in patients with fibromyalgia. *Redox Rep.* 2006;11(3):131-5

[20] Wallace DJ, Linker-Israeli M, Hallegua D, et al. Cytokines play an aetiopathogenetic role in fibromyalgia: a hypothesis and pilot study. *Rheumatology* (Oxford). 2001 Jul;40(7):743-9

[21] Pimentel M, Wallace D, Hallegua D, Chow E, Kong Y, Park S, Lin HC. A link between irritable bowel syndrome and fibromyalgia may be related to findings on lactulose breath testing. *Ann Rheum Dis.* 2004 Apr;63(4):450-2

[22] Huisman AM, White KP, Algra A, et al. Vitamin D levels in women with systemic lupus erythematosus and fibromyalgia. *J Rheumatol.* 2001 Nov;28(11):2535-9

[23] Armstrong DJ, Meenagh GK, Bickle I, Lee AS, Curran ES, Finch MB. Vitamin D deficiency is associated with anxiety and depression in fibromyalgia. *Clin Rheumatol.* 2007 Apr;26(4):551-4

[24] Hein G, Franke S. Are advanced glycation end-product-modified proteins of pathogenetic importance in fibromyalgia? *Rheumatology* (Oxford). 2002 Oct;41(10):1163-7

[25] "In the interstitial connective tissue of fibromyalgic muscles we found a more intensive staining of the AGE CML, activated NF-kappaB, and also higher CML levels in the serum of these patients compared to the controls. RAGE was only present in FM muscle." Rüster M, Franke S, Späth M, Pongratz DE, Stein G, Hein GE. Detection of elevated N epsilon-carboxymethyllysine levels in muscular tissue and in serum of patients with fibromyalgia. *Scand J Rheumatol.* 2005 Nov-Dec;34(6):460-3

[26] Simons DG, Travell JG, Simons LS. Travell & Simons' Myofascial Pain and Dysfunction. The Trigger Point Manual. Baltimore: Lippincott Williams & Wilkins; 1999

[27] Jones L, Kusunose R, Goering E. Jones Strain-Counterstrain. Carlsbad, Jones Strain Counterstrain Incorporated, 1995. [ISBN 0964513544]

[28] Hubbard DR, Berkoff GM. Myofascial trigger points show spontaneous needle EMG activity. *Spine*. 1993 Oct 1;18(13):1803-7

[29] The American College of Rheumatology 1990 Criteria for the Classification of Fibromyalgia. http://www.nfra.net/Diagnost.htm Accessed Nov 2011

[30] Wolfe F, Clauw DJ, Fitzcharles M-A, et al. The American College of Rheumatology preliminary diagnostic criteria for fibromyalgia and measurement of symptom severity. *Arthritis Care Res*. 2010;62(5):600-10 http://www.rheumatology.org/practice/clinical/classification/fibromyalgia/2010_Preliminary_Diagnostic_Criteria.pdf

[31] http://www.lilly.com/research/Pages/research.aspx and http://newsroom.lilly.com/ReleaseDetail.cfm?releaseid=316740 Accessed January 2012.

[32] Gamber RG, Shores JH, Russo DP, Jimenez C, Rubin BR. Osteopathic manipulative treatment in conjunction with medication relieves pain associated with fibromyalgia syndrome: results of a randomized clinical pilot project. *J Am Osteopath Assoc*. 2002 Jun;102(6):321-5 http://www.jaoa.org/content/102/6/321.full.pdf

[33] Leventhal LJ. Management of fibromyalgia. *Ann Intern Med*. 1999 Dec 7;131(11):850-8

[34] "Amitriptyline is a tricyclic antidepressant commonly prescribed for the treatment of several neuropathic and inflammatory illnesses. We have already reported that amitriptyline has cytotoxic effect in human cell cultures, increasing oxidative stress, and decreasing growth rate and mitochondrial activity." Bautista-Ferrufino MR, Cordero MD, Sánchez-Alcázar JA, et al. Amitriptyline induces coenzyme Q deficiency and oxidative damage in mouse lung and liver. *Toxicol Lett*. 2011 Jul 4;204(1):32-7

[35] FDA Approves First Drug for Treating Fibromyalgia. http://www.fda.gov/bbs/topics/NEWS/2007/NEW01656.html

[36] "exact mechanism of action unknown; inhibits norepinephrine and serotonin reuptake" https://online.epocrates.com; "Both Lyrica and Cymbalta reduce pain and improve function in people with fibromyalgia. While those with fibromyalgia have been shown to experience pain differently from other people, the mechanism by which these drugs produce their effects is unknown." http://www.fda.gov/ForConsumers/ConsumerUpdates/ucm107802.htm. Accessed January 2012

[37] "Internal medicine interns' perceive nutrition counseling as a priority, but lack the confidence and knowledge to effectively provide adequate nutrition education." Vetter ML, Herring SJ, Sood M, Shah NR, Kalet AL. What do resident physicians know about nutrition? An evaluation of attitudes, self-perceived proficiency and knowledge. *J Am Coll Nutr*. 2008 Apr;27(2):287-98 http://www.ncbi.nlm.nih.gov/pmc/articles/PMC2779722/

[38] "The amount of nutrition education that medical students receive continues to be inadequate." Adams KM, Kohlmeier M, Zeisel SH. Nutrition education in U.S. medical schools: latest update of a national survey. *Acad Med*. 2010 Sep;85(9):1537-42

[39] "Scientific advances on the relationship of dietary substances to the cellular mechanisms of disease occur with regularity and frequency. Yet, despite the prevalence of nutritional disorders in clinical medicine and increasing scientific evidence on the significance of dietary modification to disease prevention, present day practitioners of medicine are typically untrained in the relationship of diet to health and disease." Halsted CH. The relevance of clinical nutrition education and role models to the practice of medicine. *Eur J Clin Nutr*. 1999 May,53 Suppl 2:S29-34

[40] Vasquez A. Interventions need to be consistent with osteopathic philosophy. *J Am Osteopath Assoc*. 2006 Sep;106(9):528-9 http://www.jaoa.org/content/106/9/528.full.pdf

[41] Ely JW, Osheroff JA, Ebell MH, Bergus GR, Levy BT, Chambliss ML, Evans ER. Analysis of questions asked by family doctors regarding patient care. *BMJ*. 1999 Aug 7;319(7206):358-61 http://www.ncbi.nlm.nih.gov/pmc/articles/PMC28191/

[42] https://online.epocrates.com/noFrame/showPage.do?method=drugs&MonographId=4950 Accessed April 2012.

[43] Goldenberg DL, Burckhardt C, Crofford L. Management of fibromyalgia syndrome. *JAMA*. 2004 Nov 17;292(19):2388-95

[44] http://www.rheumatology.org/practice/clinical/patients/diseases_and_conditions/fibromyalgia.asp Accessed April 2012.

[45] American Academy of Family Physicians. http://familydoctor.org/familydoctor/en/diseases-conditions/fibromyalgia.html Accessed March 31, 2012

[46] http://www.rheumatology.org/practice/clinical/patients/diseases_and_conditions/fibromyalgia.asp Accessed March 31, 2012

[47] Plotnikoff GA, Quigley JM. Prevalence of severe hypovitaminosis D in patients with persistent, nonspecific musculoskeletal pain. *Mayo Clin Proc.* 2003;78(12):1463-70

[48] Holick MF. Vitamin D: importance in the prevention of cancers, type 1 diabetes, heart disease, and osteoporosis. *Am J Clin Nutr.* 2004 Mar;79(3):362-71

[49] Armstrong DJ, et al. Vitamin D deficiency is associated with anxiety and depression in fibromyalgia. *Clin Rheumatol.* 2007 Apr;26(4):551-4

[50] Al Faraj S, Al Mutairi K. Vitamin D deficiency and chronic low back pain in Saudi Arabia. *Spine.* 2003;28:177-9

[51] Holick MF. Vitamin D: importance in the prevention of cancers, type 1 diabetes, heart disease, and osteoporosis. *Am J Clin Nutr.* 2004 Mar;79(3):362-71

[52] Vieth R. Vitamin D supplementation, 25-hydroxyvitamin D concentrations, and safety. *Am J Clin Nutr.* 1999 May;69(5):842-56

[53] Zittermann A. Vitamin D in preventive medicine: are we ignoring the evidence? *Br J Nutr.* 2003 May;89(5):552-72

[54] Mild hypercalcemia is not necessarily a problem by itself and must be evaluated within the patient's clinical context. When blood levels of calcium (normal range: 8.7-10.4 mg/dL) reach 12.0 mg/dL patients will start to develop symptoms; with levels of 14 mg/dL or higher, the patient is generally experiencing symptoms and complications and is in need of treatment (initially with administration of intravenous fluids and a loop diuretic such as furosemide).

[55] Vieth R. Vitamin D supplementation, 25-hydroxyvitamin D concentrations, and safety. *Am J Clin Nutr.* 1999 May;69(5):842-56

[56] Vasquez A, Manso G, Cannell J. The Clinical Importance of Vitamin D (Cholecalciferol): A Paradigm Shift with Implications for All Healthcare Providers. *Alternative Therapies in Health and Medicine* 2004; 10: 28-37 http://optimalhealthresearch.com/cholecalciferol.html

[57] Vasquez A. *Musculoskeletal Pain: Expanded Clinical Strategies.* Institute for Functional Medicine. 2008

[58] Vasquez A. Revisiting the Five-Part Nutritional Wellness Protocol: The Supplemented Paleo-Mediterranean Diet. *Nutritional Perspectives* 2011 January http://optimalhealthresearch.com/protocol.html

[59] Vasquez A, Manso G, Cannell J. The Clinical Importance of Vitamin D (Cholecalciferol): A Paradigm Shift with Implications for All Healthcare Providers. *Alternative Therapies in Health and Medicine* 2004; 10: 28-37 http://optimalhealthresearch.com/cholecalciferol.html

[60] Vasquez A, Cannell J. Calcium and vitamin D in preventing fractures: data are not sufficient to show inefficacy. [letter] *BMJ: British Medical Journal* 2005;331:108-9

[61] Vasquez A. Subphysiologic Doses of Vitamin D are Subtherapeutic: Comment on the Study by The Record Trial Group. *The Lancet* 2005 Published on-line May 6 http://optimalhealthresearch.com/cholecalciferol.html

[62] Kedlaya D. Hypothyroid Myopathy. http://emedicine.medscape.com/article/313915-overview Accessed April 2012

[63] Lauritano EC, Bilotta AL, Gabrielli M, Scarpellini E, Lupascu A, Laginestra A, Novi M, Sottili S, Serricchio M, Cammarota G, Gasbarrini G, Pontecorvi A, Gasbarrini A. Association between hypothyroidism and small intestinal bacterial overgrowth. *J Clin Endocrinol Metab.* 2007 Nov;92(11):4180-4

[64] McDaniel AB. Thyroid Assessment: Controversies and Conundrums. Institute for Functional Medicine Fourteenth International Symposium. Tucson, AZ. May 23-26, 2007

[65] Friedman M, Miranda-Massari JR, Gonzalez MJ. Supraphysiological cyclic dosing of sustained release T3 in order to reset low basal body temperature. *P R Health Sci J.* 2006 Mar;25(1):23-9

[66] McDaniel AB. Thyroid Assessment: Controversies and Conundrums. Institute for Functional Medicine Fourteenth International Symposium. Tucson, AZ. May 23-26, 2007

[67] Friedman M, Miranda-Massari JR, Gonzalez MJ. Supraphysiological cyclic dosing of sustained release T3 in order to reset low basal body temperature. *P R Health Sci J.* 2006 Mar;25(1):23-9

[68] Ben-Yaakov M, Eshel G, Zaksonski L, Lazarovich Z, Boldur I. Prevalence of antibodies to Chlamydia pneumoniae in an Israeli population without clinical evidence of respiratory infection. *J Clin Pathol.* 2002 May;55(5):355-8 http://jcp.bmj.com/content/55/5/355.long

[69] Stratton C. The Role of Chlamydophila in Autoimmune Disease. 2011 International Symposium -"The Challenge of Emerging Infections in the 21st Century: Terrain, Tolerance, and Susceptibility" hosted by The Institute for Functional Medicine www.functionalmedicine.org in Seattle, Washington in May 2011

[70] "This study was a 9-month, prospective, double-blind, triple-placebo trial assessing a 6-month course of combination antibiotics as a treatment for Chlamydia-induced ReA. Groups received 1) doxycycline and rifampin plus placebo instead of azithromycin; 2) azithromycin and rifampin plus placebo instead of doxycycline; or 3) placebos instead of azithromycin, doxycycline, and rifampin. ... These data suggest that a 6-month course of combination antibiotics is an effective treatment for chronic Chlamydia-induced ReA." Carter JD, Espinoza LR, Inman RD, et al. Combination antibiotics as a treatment for chronic Chlamydia-induced reactive arthritis: a double-blind, placebo-controlled, prospective trial. *Arthritis Rheum*. 2010 May;62(5):1298-307

[71] "The frequency of Chlamydia-positive ST samples, as determined by PCR, was found to be significantly higher in patients with uSpA than in patients with OA. Our results suggest that in many patients with uSpA, chlamydial infection, which is often occult, may be the cause." Carter JD, et al. Chlamydiae as etiologic agents in chronic undifferentiated spondylarthritis. *Arthritis Rheum*. 2009 May;60(5):1311-6

[72] Appreciation is given to Bill Beakey DOM of Professional Co-Op Services http://professionalcoop.com/ for provision of this laboratory assessment.

[73] Endresen GK. Mycoplasma blood infection in chronic fatigue and fibromyalgia syndromes. *Rheumatol Int*. 2003 Sep;23(5):211-5

[74] Nicolson GL, Nasralla MY, Nicolson NL. High prevalence of Mycoplasmal infections in symptomatic (chronic fatigue syndrome) family members of *Mycoplasma*-positive Gulf War illness patients. *Journal of Chronic Fatigue Syndrome* 2003; 11(2): 21-36 http://www.immed.org/GulfWarIllness/10.01.11update/GWIfamilyJCFS_.pdf

[75] Wurapa RK, Gordeuk VR, Brittenham GM, Khiyami A, Schechter GP, Edwards CQ. Primary iron overload in African Americans. *Am J Med*. 1996 Jul;101(1):9-18

[76] Barton JC, Edwards CQ, Bertoli LF, Shroyer TW, Hudson SL. Iron overload in African Americans. *Am J Med*. 1995 Dec;99(6):616-23

[77] Vasquez A. Musculoskeletal disorders and iron overload disease: comment on the American College of Rheumatology guidelines for the initial evaluation of the adult patient with acute musculoskeletal symptoms. *Arthritis Rheum*. 1996 Oct;39(10):1767-8

[78] Barton JC, McDonnell SM, Adams PC, Brissot P, Powell LW, Edwards CQ, Cook JD, Kowdley KV. Management of hemochromatosis. Hemochromatosis Management Working Group. *Ann Intern Med*. 1998 Dec 1;129(11):932-9

[79] "However, approximately 8% of women had concentrations higher than the US Environmental Protection Agency's recom-mended reference dose (5.8 µg/L), below which exposures are considered to bewith-out adverse effects." Schober SE, et al. Blood mercury levels in US children and women of childbearing age, 1999-2000. *JAMA*. 2003 Apr 2;289(13):1667-74

[80] Kristin S. Schafer, Margaret Reeves, Skip Spitzer, Susan E. Kegley. Chemical Trespass: Pesticides in Our Bodies and Corporate Accountability. Pesticide Action Network North America. May 2004 Available at http://www.panna.org/campaigns/docsTrespass/chemicalTrespass2004.dv.html on August 1, 2004 See also: Body Burden: The Pollution in People. http://ewg.org/issues/siteindex/issues.php?issueid=5004 Accessed February 6, 2006

[81] Crinnion WJ. Environmental medicine, part one: the human burden of environmental toxins and their common health effects. *Altern Med Rev*. 2000 Feb;5(1):52-63

[82] Crinnion WJ. Environmental medicine, part 2 - health effects of and protection from ubiquitous airborne solvent exposure. *Altern Med Rev*. 2000 Apr;5(2):133-43

[83] Crinnion WJ. Environmental medicine, part three: long-term effects of chronic low-dose mercury exposure. *Altern Med Rev*. 2000 Jun;5(3):209-23

[84] Crinnion WJ. Environmental medicine, part 4: pesticides - biologically persistent and ubiquitous toxins. *Altern Med Rev*. 2000 Oct;5(5):432-47

[85] Elemental Mercury Vapor Poisoning -- North Carolina, 1988. http://www.cdc.gov/mmwr/preview/mmwrhtml/00001499.htm

[86] Shih H, Gartner JC Jr. Weight loss, hypertension, weakness, and limb pain in an 11-year-old boy. *J Pediatr*. 2001 Apr;138(4):566-9

[87] Sterzl I, Prochazkova J, Hrda P, Bartova J, Matucha P, Stejskal VD. Mercury and nickel allergy: risk factors in fatigue and autoimmunity. *Neuro Endocrinol Lett*. 1999;20:221-8

[88] Padlewska KK. Acrodynia. Last Updated: February 15, 2007 eMedicine http://www.emedicine.com/derm/topic592.htm Accessed October 25, 2007

[89] Chugh KS, Singhal PC, Uberoi HS. Rhabdomyolysis and renal failure in acute mercuric chloride poisoning. *Med J Aust*. 1978 Jul 29;2(3):125-6

[90] Chiu VC, Mouring D, Haynes DH. Action of mercurials on the active and passive transport properties of sarcoplasmic reticulum. *J Bioenerg Biomembr*. 1983 Feb;15(1):13-25

[91] Shamoo AE, Maclennan DH, Elderfrawi ME. Differential effects of mercurial compounds on excitable tissues. *Chem Biol Interact.* 1976 Jan;12(1):41-52

[92] Kalra V, Dua T, Kumar V, Kaul B. Succimer in Symptomatic Lead Poisoning. *Indian Pediatrics* 2002; 39:580-585 http://www.indianpediatrics.net/june2002/june-580-585.htm

[93] Bradstreet J, Geier DA, Kartzinel JJ, Adams JB, Geier MR. A case-control study of mercury burden in children with autistic spectrum disorders. *Journal of American Physicians and Surgeons* 2003; 8: 76-79 http://www.jpands.org/vol8no3/geier.pdf

[94] Forman J, Moline J, Cernichiari E, Sayegh S, Torres JC, Landrigan MM, Hudson J, Adel HN, Landrigan PJ. A cluster of pediatric metallic mercury exposure cases treated with meso-2,3-dimercaptosuccinic acid (DMSA). *Environ Health Perspect.* 2000 Jun;108(6):575-7 http://ehp.niehs.nih.gov/docs/2000/108p575-577forman/abstract.html

[95] Miller AL. Dimercaptosuccinic acid (DMSA), a non-toxic, water-soluble treatment for heavy metal toxicity. *Altern Med Rev.* 1998 Jun;3(3):199-207

[96] Kotter I, Durk H, Saal JG, Kroiher A, Schweinsberg F. Mercury exposure from dental amalgam fillings in the etiology of primary fibromyalgia: a pilot study. *J Rheumatol.* 1995 Nov;22(11):2194-5

[97] Cobbett CS. Phytochelatins and their roles in heavy metal detoxification. *Plant Physiol.* 2000;123:825-32 plantphysiol.org/content/123/3/825

[98] Vasquez A. *Musculoskeletal Pain: Expanded Clinical Strategies*: published in 2008 by the Institute for Functional Medicine www.FunctionalMedicine.org

[99] Sverdrup B. Use less cosmetics--suffer less from fibromyalgia? *J Womens Health* (Larchmt). 2004 Mar;13(2):187-94

[100] Crinnion WJ. Environmental medicine, part three: long-term effects of chronic low-dose mercury exposure. *Altern Med Rev.* 2000 Jun;5(3):209-23 http://www.thorne.com/altmedrev/.fulltext/5/3/209.pdf

[101] "The Food and Drug Administration has recently licensed the drug DMSA (succimer) for reduction of blood lead levels >/= 45 micrograms/dl. This decision was based on the demonstrated ability of DMSA to reduce blood lead levels. An advantage of this drug is that it can be given orally." Goyer RA, Cherian MG, Jones MM, Reigart JR. Role of chelating agents for prevention, intervention, and treatment of exposures to toxic metals. *Environ Health Perspect.* 1995 Nov;103(11):1048-52 Http://ehp.niehs.nih.gov/docs/1995/103-11/meetingreport.html

[102] Bradstreet J, Geier DA, Kartzinel JJ, Adams JB, Geier MR. A case-control study of mercury burden in children with autistic spectrum disorders. *Journal of American Physicians and Surgeons* 2003; 8: 76-79 http://www.jpands.org/vol8no3/geier.pdf

[103] Crinnion WJ. Environmental medicine, part three: long-term effects of chronic low-dose mercury exposure. *Altern Med Rev.* 2000 Jun;5(3):209-23

[104] Forman J, Moline J, Cernichiari E, Sayegh S, Torres JC, Landrigan MM, Hudson J, Adel HN, Landrigan PJ. A cluster of pediatric metallic mercury exposure cases treated with meso-2,3-dimercaptosuccinic acid (DMSA). *Environ Health Perspect.* 2000 Jun;108(6):575-7 http://ehp.niehs.nih.gov/docs/2000/108p575-577forman/abstract.html

[105] Miller AL. Dimercaptosuccinic acid (DMSA), a non-toxic, water-soluble treatment for heavy metal toxicity. *Altern Med Rev.* 1998 Jun;3(3):199-207 http://www.thorne.com/altmedrev/.fulltext/3/3/199.pdf

[106] DMSA. *Altern Med Rev.* 2000 Jun;5(3):264-7 http://thorne.com/altmedrev/.fulltext/5/3/264.pdf

[107] Vasquez A. *Integrative Rheumatology.* IBMRC 2006, 2007 and all future editions. http://optimalhealthresearch.com/rheumatology.html

[108] Vasquez A. *Musculoskeletal Pain: Expanded Clinical Strategies.* Institute for Functional Medicine. 2008

[109] Vasquez A. *Musculoskeletal Pain: Expanded Clinical Strategies.* Institute for Functional Medicine. 2008

[110] Pimentel M, Wallace D, Hallegua D, Chow E, Kong Y, Park S, Lin HC. A link between irritable bowel syndrome and fibromyalgia may be related to findings on lactulose breath testing. *Ann Rheum Dis.* 2004 Apr;63(4):450-2

[111] Lubrano E, et al. Fibromyalgia in patients with irritable bowel syndrome. An association with the severity of the intestinal disorder. *Int J Colorectal Dis.* 2001 Aug;16(4):211-5

[112] Veale D, Kavanagh G, Fielding JF, Fitzgerald O. Primary fibromyalgia and the irritable bowel syndrome: different expressions of a common pathogenetic process. *Br J Rheumatol.* 1991 Jun;30(3):220-2

[113] Lin HC. Small intestinal bacterial overgrowth: a framework for understanding irritable bowel syndrome. *JAMA.* 2004 Aug 18;292(7):852-8

[114] Pimentel M, Wallace D, Hallegua D, Chow E, Kong Y, Park S, Lin HC. A link between irritable bowel syndrome and fibromyalgia may be related to findings on lactulose breath testing. *Ann Rheum Dis.* 2004 Apr;63(4):450-2

[115] Bundgaard H, Kjeldsen K, Suarez Krabbe K, van Hall G, Simonsen L, Qvist J, Hansen CM, Moller K, Fonsmark L, Lav Madsen P, Klarlund Pedersen B. Endotoxemia stimulates skeletal muscle Na+-K+-ATPase and raises blood lactate under aerobic conditions in humans. *Am J Physiol Heart Circ Physiol.* 2003 Mar;284(3):H1028-34

[116] Vella A, Farrugia G. D-lactic acidosis: pathologic consequence of saprophytism. *Mayo Clin Proc.* 1998 May;73(5):451-6

[117] Attene-Ramos MS, Wagner ED, Gaskins HR, Plewa MJ. Hydrogen sulfide induces direct radical-associated DNA damage. *Mol Cancer Res.* 2007 May;5(5):455-9

[118] Magee EA, Richardson CJ, Hughes R, Cummings JH. Contribution of dietary protein to sulfide production in the large intestine: an in vitro and a controlled feeding study in humans. *Am J Clin Nutr.* 2000 Dec;72(6):1488-94

[119] Babidge W, Millard S, Roediger W. Sulfides impair short chain fatty acid beta-oxidation at acyl-CoA dehydrogenase level in colonocytes: implications for ulcerative colitis. *Mol Cell Biochem.* 1998 Apr;181(1-2):117-24

[120] Lemle MD. Hypothesis: chronic fatigue syndrome is caused by dysregulation of hydrogen sulfide metabolism. *Med Hypotheses.* 2009 Jan;72(1):108-9

[121] White RR 4th, Mela L, Miller LD, Berwick L. Effect of E. coli endotoxin on mitochondrial form and function: inability to complete succinate-induced condensed-to-orthodox conformational change. *Ann Surg.* 1971 Dec;174(6):983-90

[122] Sheedy JR, Wettenhall RE, Scanlon D, Gooley PR, Lewis DP, McGregor N, Stapleton DI, Butt HL, DE Meirleir KL. Increased d-lactic acid intestinal bacteria in patients with chronic fatigue syndrome. *In Vivo.* 2009 Jul-Aug;23(4):621-8

[123] Lin HC. Small intestinal bacterial overgrowth: a framework for understanding irritable bowel syndrome. *JAMA.* 2004 Aug 18;292(7):852-8

[124] Othman M, Agüero R, Lin HC. Alterations in intestinal microbial flora and human disease. *Curr Opin Gastroenterol.* 2008 Jan;24(1):11-6

[125] Meeus M, Nijs J. Central sensitization: a biopsychosocial explanation for chronic widespread pain in patients with fibromyalgia and chronic fatigue syndrome. *Clin Rheumatol.* 2007 Apr;26(4):465-73

[126] Johnston IN, Westbrook RF. Inhibition of morphine analgesia by LPS: role of opioid and NMDA receptors and spinal glia. *Behav Brain Res.* 2005;156(1):75-83

[127] Othman M, Agüero R, Lin HC. Alterations in intestinal microbial flora and human disease. *Curr Opin Gastroenterol.* 2008 Jan;24(1):11-6

[128] Elphick HL, Elphick DA, Sanders DS. Small bowel bacterial overgrowth. An underrecognized cause of malnutrition in older adults. Geriatrics. 2006 Sep;61(9):21-6

[129] McEvoy A, Dutton J, James OF. Bacterial contamination of the small intestine is an important cause of occult malabsorption in the elderly. *Br Med J* (Clin Res Ed). 1983 Sep 17;287(6395):789-93 http://www.ncbi.nlm.nih.gov/pmc/articles/PMC1549133/

[130] Cordero MD, De Miguel M, Moreno Fernández AM, et al. Mitochondrial dysfunction and mitophagy activation in blood mononuclear cells of fibromyalgia patients: implications in the pathogenesis of the disease. *Arthritis Res Ther.* 2010;12(1):R17

[131] Wang ZQ, Porreca F, Cuzzocrea S, Galen K, Lightfoot R, Masini E, Muscoli C, Mollace V, Ndengele M, Ischiropoulos H, Salvemini D. A newly identified role for superoxide in inflammatory pain. *J Pharmacol Exp Ther.* 2004 Jun;309(3):869-78

[132] Ilnytska O, Lyzogubov VV, Stevens MJ, Drel VR, Mashtalir N, Pacher P, Yorek MA, Obrosova IG. Poly(ADP-ribose) polymerase inhibition alleviates experimental diabetic sensory neuropathy. *Diabetes.* 2006 Jun;55(6):1686-94

[133] "Plasma-free tryptophan is inversely related to the severity of subjective pain in 8 patients who fulfilled criteria for a variety of non-articular rheumatism, the "fibrositis syndrome". The observation is consistent with animal and human studies suggesting a relationship between reduced brain serotonin metabolism and pain reactivity." Moldofsky H, Warsh JJ. Plasma tryptophan and musculoskeletal pain in non-articular rheumatism ("fibrositis syndrome"). *Pain.* 1978 Jun;5(1):65-71

[134] Demoss RD, Moser K. Tryptophanase in Diverse Bacterial Species. *Journal of Bacteriology* 1969; 98: 167-171

[135] "A strong negative correlation between SP and 5-HIAA (P = .000) as well as between SP and TRP (P = .009) could be demonstrated. High serum concentrations of 5-HIAA and TRP showed a significant relation to low pain scores (5-HIAA: P = .030; TRP: P = .014). Moreover, 5-HIAA was strongly related to good quality of sleep (P = .000), while SP was related to sleep disturbance (P = .005)." Schwarz MJ, Späth M, Müller-Bardorff H, Pongratz DE, Bondy B, Ackenheil M. Relationship of substance P, 5-

hydroxyindole acetic acid and tryptophan in serum of fibromyalgia patients. *Neurosci Lett.* 1999 Jan 15;259(3):196-8

[136] "The FMS patients had a 31% lower MT secretion than healthy subjects during the hours of darkness... Patients with fibromyalgic syndrome have a lower melatonin secretion during the hours of darkness than healthy subjects. This may contribute to impaired sleep at night, fatigue during the day, and changed pain perception." Wikner J, Hirsch U, Wetterberg L, Röjdmark S. Fibromyalgia--a syndrome associated with decreased nocturnal melatonin secretion. *Clin Endocrinol* (Oxf). 1998 Aug;49(2):179-83

[137] Weinstock LB, Fern SE, Duntley SP. Restless Legs Syndrome in Patients with Irritable Bowel Syndrome: Response to Small Intestinal Bacterial Overgrowth Therapy. *Dig Dis Sci.* 2007 May;53(5):1252-6

[138] Wallace DJ, Hallegua DS. Fibromyalgia: the gastrointestinal link. *Curr Pain Headache Rep.* 2004 Oct;8(5):364-8

[139] Pimentel M, Hallegua DS, Wallace DJ, et al.: Improvement of symptoms by eradication of small intestinal overgrowth in FM: a double-blind study. [Abstract] *Arthritis Rheum* 1999, 42:S343

[140] Pimentel M, Park S, Mirocha J, Kane SV, Kong Y. The effect of a nonabsorbed oral antibiotic (rifaximin) on the symptoms of the irritable bowel syndrome: a randomized trial. *Ann Intern Med.* 2006 Oct 17;145(8):557-63

[141] Sharara AI, Aoun E, Abdul-Baki H, Mounzer R, Sidani S, Elhajj I. A randomized double-blind placebo-controlled trial of rifaximin in patients with abdominal bloating and flatulence. *Am J Gastroenterol.* 2006 Feb;101(2):326-33

[142] Pimentel M, Lembo A, Chey WD, et al. Rifaximin therapy for patients with irritable bowel syndrome without constipation. *N Engl J Med.* 2011 Jan 6;364(1):22-32

[143] Pimentel M. Review of rifaximin as treatment for SIBO and IBS. *Expert Opin Investig Drugs.* 2009 Mar;18(3):349-58

[144] Wallace DJ, Hallegua DS. Fibromyalgia: the gastrointestinal link. *Curr Pain Headache Rep.* 2004 Oct;8(5):364-8

[145] Shedlofsky SI, Israel BC, McClain CJ, Hill DB, Blouin RA. Endotoxin administration to humans inhibits hepatic cytochrome P450-mediated drug metabolism. *J Clin Invest.* 1994 Dec;94(6):2209-14

[146] Dunstan RH, Donohoe M, Taylor W, Roberts TK, Murdoch RN, Watkins JA, McGregor NR. A preliminary investigation of chlorinated hydrocarbons and chronic fatigue syndrome. *Med J Aust.* 1995 Sep 18;163(6):294-7

[147] Malik BA, Xie YY, Wine E, Huynh HQ. Diagnosis and pharmacological management of small intestinal bacterial overgrowth in children with intestinal failure. *Can J Gastroenterol.* 2011 Jan;25(1):41-5. This is a remarkable article and probably one of the most brilliant articles on the treatment of SIBO with drugs.

[148] [No authors listed] Berberine. *Altern Med Rev.* 2000 Apr;5(2):175-7

[149] "A case report of a patient with SIBO who showed marked subjective improvement in IBS-like symptoms and significant reductions in hydrogen production after treatment with ECPO is presented. While further investigation is necessary, the results in this case suggest one of the mechanisms by which ECPO improves IBS symptoms is antimicrobial activity in the small intestine." Logan AC, Beaulne TM. The treatment of small intestinal bacterial overgrowth with enteric-coated peppermint oil: a case report. *Altern Med Rev.* 2002 Oct;7(5):410-7

[150] Force M, Sparks WS, Ronzio RA. Inhibition of enteric parasites by emulsified oil of oregano in vivo. *Phytother Res.* 2000 May;14(3):213-4

[151] Vasquez A. Reducing Pain and Inflammation Naturally. Part 6: Nutritional and Botanical Treatments Against "Silent Infections" and Gastrointestinal Dysbiosis, Commonly Overlooked Causes of Neuromusculoskeletal Inflammation and Chronic Health Problems. *Nutr Perspect* 2006; Jan: 5-21. For more updated information, see: Vasquez A. *Integrative Rheumatology.* Integrative and Biological Medicine Research and Consulting. http://optimalhealthresearch.com/textbooks/rheumatology.html

[152] Milanski M, et al. Saturated fatty acids produce an inflammatory response predominantly through the activation of TLR4 signaling in hypothalamus: implications for the pathogenesis of obesity. *J Neurosci.* 2009 Jan 14;29(2):359-70

[153] Because the kidneys are responsible for excreting potassium, reduced kidney function (kidney failure, renal insufficiency) implies that the kidneys may not be able to perform the function of excreting potassium; thus, consumption of a potassium-rich diet could contribute to a dangerous situation of excess potassium in the blood known as hyperkalemia (*hyper*=too much, *kal*=potassium, *emia*=blood disorder). For patients with renal insufficiency, consumption of an otherwise health-promoting diet rich in fruits and vegetables might cause a problem if potassium accumulates in the blood due to impaired excretion. Blood tests can assess renal function as well as the blood potassium level. This is one example of why a

clinician/doctor should be employed by patients before implementing diet modification and nutritional supplementation. Dr Vasquez can be contacted via his websites http://HealGrowThriveMedicine.com/ (for patients) and http://OptimalHealthResearch.com/ (for doctors and students).

[154] "The modern Western-type diet is deficient in fruits and vegetables and contains excessive animal products, generating the accumulation of non-metabolizable anions and a lifespan state of overlooked metabolic acidosis, whose magnitude increases progressively with aging due to the physiological decline in kidney function." Adeva MM, Souto G. Diet-induced metabolic acidosis. *Clin Nutr.* 2011 Aug;30(4):416-21

[155] Donaldson MS, Speight N, Loomis S. Fibromyalgia syndrome improved using a mostly raw vegetarian diet: an observational study. *BMC Complement Altern Med.* 2001;1:7 http://www.biomedcentral.com/1472-6882/1/7

[156] Michalsen A, Riegert M, Lüdtke R, Bäcker M, Langhorst J, Schwickert M, Dobos GJ. Mediterranean diet or extended fasting's influence on changing the intestinal microflora, immunoglobulin A secretion and clinical outcome in patients with rheumatoid arthritis and fibromyalgia: an observational study. *BMC Complement Altern Med.* 2005 Dec 22;5:22

[157] "In the interstitial connective tissue of fibromyalgic muscles we found a more intensive staining of the AGE CML, activated NF-kappaB, and also higher CML levels in the serum of these patients compared to the controls. RAGE was only present in FM muscle." Rüster M, Franke S, Späth M, Pongratz DE, Stein G, Hein GE. Detection of elevated N epsilon-carboxymethyllysine levels in muscular tissue and in serum of patients with fibromyalgia. *Scand J Rheumatol.* 2005 Nov-Dec;34(6):460-3

[158] Gaby AR. The role of Coenzyme Q10 in clinical medicine: Part 1. *Altern Med Rev* 1996;1:11-17

[159] Gaby AR. The role of Coenzyme Q10 in clinical medicine: Part 2. *Altern Med Rev* 1996;1: 168-175

[160] Cordero MD, De Miguel M, Moreno Fernández AM, et al. Mitochondrial dysfunction and mitophagy activation in blood mononuclear cells of fibromyalgia patients: implications in the pathogenesis of the disease. *Arthritis Res Ther.* 2010;12(1):R17. Epub 2010 Jan 28.

[161] Cordero MD, De Miguel M, Moreno Fernández AM, Carmona López IM, Garrido Maraver J, Cotán D, Gómez Izquierdo L, Bonal P, Campa F, Bullon P, Navas P, Sánchez Alcázar JA. Mitochondrial dysfunction and mitophagy activation in blood mononuclear cells of fibromyalgia patients: implications in the pathogenesis of the disease. *Arthritis Res Ther.* 2010;12(1):R17. Epub 2010 Jan 28.

[162] Lister RE. An open, pilot study to evaluate the potential benefits of coenzyme Q10 combined with Ginkgo biloba extract in fibromyalgia syndrome. *J Int Med Res.* 2002 Mar-Apr;30(2):195-9

[163] Cordero MD et al. Coenzyme Q(10): a novel therapeutic approach for Fibromyalgia? case series with 5 patients. *Mitochondrion.* 2011 Jul;11(4):623-5

[164] Cordero MD, Cano-García FJ, Alcocer-Gómez E, et al. Oxidative stress correlates with headache symptoms in fibromyalgia: coenzyme Q_{10} effect on clinical improvement. *PLoS One.* 2012;7(4):e35677 http://www.ncbi.nlm.nih.gov/pmc/articles/PMC3330812/

[165] Moldofsky H, Warsh JJ. Plasma tryptophan and musculoskeletal pain in non-articular rheumatism ("fibrositis syndrome"). *Pain.* 1978 Jun;5(1):65-71

[166] Yunus MB, Dailey JW, Aldag JC, Masi AT, Jobe PC. Plasma tryptophan and other amino acids in primary fibromyalgia: a controlled study. *J Rheumatol.* 1992 Jan;19(1):90-4

[167] Russell IJ, Michalek JE, Vipraio GA, Fletcher EM, Wall K. Serum amino acids in fibrositis/fibromyalgia syndrome. *J Rheumatol Suppl.* 1989 Nov;19:158-63

[168] Wolfe F, Russell IJ, Vipraio G, Ross K, Anderson J. Serotonin levels, pain threshold, and fibromyalgia symptoms in the general population. J Rheumatol. 1997;24(3):555-9

[169] Caruso I, Sarzi Puttini P, Cazzola M, Azzolini V. Double-blind study of 5-hydroxytryptophan versus placebo in the treatment of primary fibromyalgia syndrome. *J Int Med Res.* 1990 May-Jun;18(3):201-9

[170] Sarzi Puttini P, Caruso I. Primary fibromyalgia syndrome and 5-hydroxy-L-tryptophan: a 90-day open study. *J Int Med Res.* 1992 Apr;20(2):182-9

[171] Caruso I, Sarzi Puttini P, Cazzola M, Azzolini V. Double-blind study of 5-hydroxytryptophan versus placebo in the treatment of primary fibromyalgia syndrome. *J Int Med Res.* 1990 May-Jun;18(3):201-9

[172] Wikner J, et al. Fibromyalgia--a syndrome associated with decreased nocturnal melatonin secretion. *Clin Endocrinol* (Oxf). 1998 Aug;49(2):179-83

[173] León J, Acuña-Castroviejo D, Escames G, Tan DX, Reiter RJ. Melatonin mitigates mitochondrial malfunction. *J Pineal Res.* 2005 Jan;38(1):1-9

[174] Acuna-Castroviejo D, Escames G, Reiter RJ. Melatonin therapy in fibromyalgia. *J Pineal Res.* 2006 Jan;40(1):98-9

[175] Hussain SA, Al-Khalifa II, Jasim NA, Gorial FI. Adjuvant use of melatonin for treatment of fibromyalgia. *J Pineal Res.* 2011 Apr;50(3):267-71

[176] Cordain L, Eaton SB, Sebastian A, Mann N, Lindeberg S, Watkins BA, O'Keefe JH, Brand-Miller J. Origins and evolution of the Western diet: health implications for the 21st century. *Am J Clin Nutr.* 2005 Feb;81(2):341-54

[177] Rylander R, Remer T, Berkemeyer S, Vormann J. Acid-base status affects renal magnesium losses in healthy, elderly persons. *J Nutr.* 2006 Sep;136(9):2374-7

[178] Russell IJ, Michalek JE, Flechas JD, Abraham GE. Treatment of fibromyalgia syndrome with Super Malic: a randomized, double blind, placebo controlled, crossover pilot study. *J Rheumatol.* 1995 May;22(5):953-8

[179] Rossini M, Di Munno O, Valentini G, Bianchi G, Biasi G, Cacace E, Malesci D, La Montagna G, Viapiana O, Adami S. Double-blind, multicenter trial comparing acetyl l-carnitine with placebo in the treatment of fibromyalgia patients. *Clin Exp Rheumatol.* 2007 Mar-Apr;25(2):182-8

[180] Teitelbaum JE, Johnson C, St Cyr J. The use of D-ribose in chronic fatigue syndrome and fibromyalgia: a pilot study. *J Altern Complement Med.* 2006 Nov;12(9):857-62

[181] Amital D, Vishne T, Rubinow A, Levine J. Observed effects of creatine monohydrate in a patient with depression and fibromyalgia. *Am J Psychiatry.* 2006 Oct;163(10):1840-1

[182] Watanabe A, Kato N, Kato T. Effects of creatine on mental fatigue and cerebral hemoglobin oxygenation. *Neurosci Res.* 2002 Apr;42(4):279-85

[183] Citak-Karakaya I, Akbayrak T, Demirturk F, Ekici G, Bakar Y. Short and long-term results of connective tissue manipulation and combined ultrasound therapy in patients with fibromyalgia. *J Manipulative Physiol Ther.* 2006 Sep;29(7):524-8

[184] Blunt KL, Rajwani MH, Guerriero RC. The effectiveness of chiropractic management of fibromyalgia patients: a pilot study. *J Manipulative Physiol Ther.* 1997 Jul-Aug;20(6):389-99

[185] Martin DP, Sletten CD, Williams BA, Berger IH. Improvement in fibromyalgia symptoms with acupuncture: results of a randomized controlled trial. *Mayo Clin Proc.* 2006 Jun;81(6):749-57

[186] Singh BB, Wu WS, Hwang SH, Khorsan R, Der-Martirosian C, Vinjamury SP, Wang CN, Lin SY. Effectiveness of acupuncture in the treatment of fibromyalgia. *Altern Ther Health Med.* 2006 Mar-Apr;12(2):34-41

[187] Deluze C, Bosia L, Zirbs A, Chantraine A, Vischer TL. Electroacupuncture in fibromyalgia: results of a controlled trial. *BMJ.* 1992 Nov 21;305(6864):1249-52

[188] Sandberg M, Larsson B, Lindberg LG, Gerdle B. Different patterns of blood flow response in the trapezius muscle following needle stimulation (acupuncture) between healthy subjects and patients with fibromyalgia and work-related trapezius myalgia. *Eur J Pain.* 2005 Oct;9(5):497-510

[189] Sandberg M, Lindberg LG, Gerdle B. Peripheral effects of needle stimulation (acupuncture) on skin and muscle blood flow in fibromyalgia. *Eur J Pain.* 2004 Apr;8(2):163-71

[190] Harris RE, Tian X, Williams DA, Tian TX, Cupps TR, Petzke F, Groner KH, Biswas P, Gracely RH, Clauw DJ. Treatment of fibromyalgia with formula acupuncture: investigation of needle placement, needle stimulation, and treatment frequency. *J Altern Complement Med.* 2005 Aug;11(4):663-71

[191] Assefi NP, Sherman KJ, Jacobsen C, Goldberg J, Smith WR, Buchwald D.A randomized clinical trial of acupuncture compared with sham acupuncture in fibromyalgia. *Ann Intern Med.* 2005 Jul 5;143(1):10-9

[192] Mein EA, Greenman PE, McMillin DL, Richards DG, Nelson CD. Manual medicine diversity: research pitfalls and the emerging medical paradigm. *J Am Osteopath Assoc.* 2001 Aug;101(8):441-4

[193] Gamber RG, Shores JH, Russo DP, Jimenez C, Rubin BR. Osteopathic manipulative treatment in conjunction with medication relieves pain associated with fibromyalgia syndrome: results of a randomized clinical pilot project. *J Am Osteopath Assoc.* 2002 Jun;102(6):321-5

[194] Chen KW, Hassett AL, Hou F, Staller J, Lichtbroun AS.A pilot study of external qigong therapy for patients with fibromyalgia. *J Altern Complement Med.* 2006 Nov;12(9):851-6

[195] Ardiç F, Ozgen M, Aybek H, Rota S, Cubukçu D, Gökgöz A. Effects of balneotherapy on serum IL-1, PGE2 and LTB4 levels in fibromyalgia patients. *Rheumatol Int.* 2007 Mar;27(5):441-6

[196] Evcik D, Kizilay B, Gökçen E. The effects of balneotherapy on fibromyalgia patients. *Rheumatol Int.* 2002 Jun;22(2):56-9

[197] Fioravanti A, Perpignano G, Tirri G, Cardinale G, Gianniti C, Lanza CE, Loi A, Tirri E, Sfriso P, Cozzi F. Effects of mud-bath treatment on fibromyalgia patients: a randomized clinical trial. *Rheumatol Int.* 2007 Oct;27(12):1157-61

[198] Dönmez A, Karagülle MZ, Tercan N, Dinler M, Işsever H, Karagülle M, Turan M. SPA therapy in fibromyalgia: a randomised controlled clinic study. *Rheumatol Int.* 2005 Dec;26(2):168-72

[199] Leventhal LJ. Management of fibromyalgia. *Ann Intern Med.* 1999 Dec 7;131(11):850-8

[200] Merchant RE, Carmack CA, Wise CM. Nutritional supplementation with Chlorella pyrenoidosa for patients with fibromyalgia syndrome: a pilot study. *Phytother Res.* 2000 May;14(3):167-73

[201] Pore RS. Detoxification of chlordecone poisoned rats with chlorella and chlorella derived sporopollenin. *Drug Chem Toxicol.* 1984;7(1):57-71

[202] Morita K, Ogata M, Hasegawa T. Chlorophyll derived from Chlorella inhibits dioxin absorption from the gastrointestinal tract and accelerates dioxin excretion in rats. *Environ Health Perspect.* 2001 Mar;109(3):289-94

[203] Morita K, Matsueda T, Iida T, Hasegawa T. Chlorella accelerates dioxin excretion in rats. *J Nutr.* 1999 Sep;129(9):1731-6

[204] Nakano S, Noguchi T, Takekoshi H, Suzuki G, Nakano M. Maternal-fetal distribution and transfer of dioxins in pregnant women in Japan, and attempts to reduce maternal transfer with Chlorella (Chlorella pyrenoidosa) supplements. *Chemosphere.* 2005 Dec;61(9):1244-55

[205] Nakano S, Takekoshi H, Nakano M. Chlorella (Chlorella pyrenoidosa) supplementation decreases dioxin and increases immunoglobulin a concentrations in breast milk. *J Med Food.* 2007 Mar;10(1):134-42

[206] Quigley EM, Flourie B. Probiotics and irritable bowel syndrome: a rationale for their use and an assessment of the evidence to date. *Neurogastroenterol Motil.* 2007 Mar;19(3):166-72

[207] O'Mahony L, McCarthy J, Kelly P, Hurley G, Luo F, Chen K, O'Sullivan GC, Kiely B, Collins JK, Shanahan F, Quigley EM. Lactobacillus and bifidobacterium in irritable bowel syndrome: symptom responses and relationship to cytokine profiles. *Gastroenterology.* 2005 Mar;128(3):541-51

[208] Shornikova AV, Casas IA, Mykkänen H, Salo E, Vesikari T. Bacteriotherapy with Lactobacillus reuteri in rotavirus gastroenteritis. *Pediatr Infect Dis J.* 1997 ;16(12):1103-7

[209] Rosenfeldt V, Benfeldt E, Valerius NH, Paerregaard A, Michaelsen KF. Effect of probiotics on gastrointestinal symptoms and small intestinal permeability in children with atopic dermatitis. *J Pediatr.* 2004 Nov;145(5):612-6

[210] Simenhoff ML, Dunn SR, Zollner GP, Fitzpatrick ME, Emery SM, Sandine WE, Ayres JW. Biomodulation of the toxic and nutritional effects of small bowel bacterial overgrowth in end-stage kidney disease using freeze-dried Lactobacillus acidophilus. *Miner Electrolyte Metab.* 1996;22(1-3):92-6

[211] **Vasquez A**. Zinc treatment for reduction of hyperplasia of prostate. *Townsend Letter for Doctors and Patients* 1996; January: 100

[212] Broad W, Wade N. *Betrayers of the Truth: Fraud and Deceit in the Halls of Science*. New York: Simon and Schuster; 1982

[213] Davies R. *Reading and Writing*. Salt Lake City: University of Utah Press; 1992, page 23

[214] Dr Vasquez's perspective: I have trained in functional medicine since 1994, first as a student of Jeffrey Bland PhD *et al* and later as Forum Consultant and Faculty (2003 – present in 2011) for the Institute of Functional Medicine, and I wrote three chapters in *Textbook of Functional Medicine* published by Institute of Functional Medicine. My opinions here are not necessarily currently representative of the Institute of Functional Medicine in this context.

[215] **Vasquez A**. Web-like Interconnections of Physiological Factors. *Integrative Medicine: A Clinician's Journal* 2006, April/May, 32-37

Made in the USA
San Bernardino, CA
27 August 2013